ALL NEW

EASY
LOW-CARB
COOKING

Published by ECW Press
2120 Queen Street East, Suite 200, Toronto, Ontario, Canada M4E 1E2

NATIONAL LIBRARY OF CANADA CATALOGUING IN PUBLICATION

Haakonson, Patricia, 1950–
All new easy low-carb cooking : over 300 delicious recipes including breads, muffins, cookies
and desserts / Patricia Haakonson.

ISBN 1-55022-681-9

1. Complex carbohydrate diet — Recipes. I. Title.

RM222.2.H32 2004   641.5'638   C2004-902609-7

Editing: Joy Gugeler
Cover photo: Michael Tourigny
Cover and Text Design: Tania Craan
Typesetting: Mary Bowness
Printing: Webcom

This book is set in AGaramond.

The publication of *All New Easy Low-Carb Cooking* has been generously supported
by the Canada Council, the Ontario Arts Council, the Government
of Canada through the Book Publishing Industry
Development Program. **Canada**

DISTRIBUTION
CANADA: Jaguar Book Group, 100 Armstrong Avenue, Georgetown, ON, L7G 5S4
UNITED STATES: Independent Publishers Group, 814 North Franklin Street,
Chicago, Illinois 60610

PRINTED AND BOUND IN CANADA

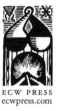

ECW PRESS
ecwpress.com

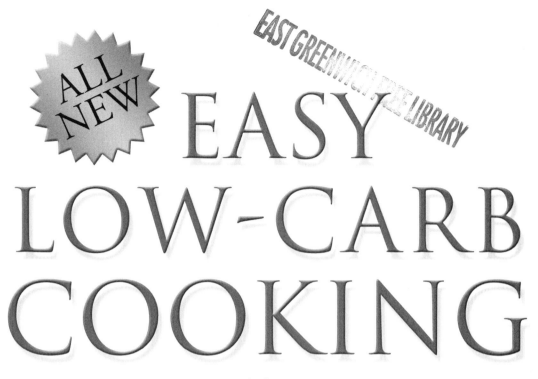

ALL NEW EASY LOW-CARB COOKING

Over 300 delicious recipes
including breads, muffins, cookies and desserts

PATRICIA HAAKONSON, B.SC.

ECW PRESS

Contents

SALADS   85

SALAD DRESSINGS & SAUCES   115

FISH   231

MEATS   249

COOKIES   293

DESSERTS   305

Introduction

Five years ago my life took a dramatic turn when I decided to try a moderated low-carb diet to lose some weight. I chose a plan similar to the widely known Dr. Atkins' (Low Carbohydrate) Diet. There are many diets that employ the same basic principles, including *The Protein Power Lifeplan, The Sugar Busters Diet, The Carbohydrate Addict's Diet, The Zone,* and *The South Beach Diet.* Like many other people, I had gained and lost weight many times in my adult life but had not been successful in keeping the weight off. I was determined that this time would be different.

The basic principle of any low-carbohydrate diet is simple. The body, in order to create energy, will burn either fat or sugar for fuel. By reducing the amount of carbohydrate we ingest (which the body converts to sugar for energy), we force the body to burn fat for energy. Then, if we consume less fat than we need to maintain our activity level, we will actually burn the fat that our bodies have stored over the years. During maintenance, we can increase the amount of carbohydrate because we are no longer concerned with burning stored fat. As with any weight loss or weight management program, moderate exercise on a regular basis will improve overall health and well-being.

I was skeptical about this approach to eating and weight loss and worried that I would not be able to stick to the stringent requirement to give up my beloved breads, bagels, potatoes, and pasta. I had adopted a diet that was very high in carbohydrate in my efforts to reduce my fat intake. What I unwittingly did was sabotage my efforts to be healthy. I was overproducing insulin. This resulted in loss of energy and periods of lethargy induced by insulin highs and blood sugar lows.

Adhering to my eating plan turned out to be a lot easier than I had anticipated. To my delight, I lost more than 40 pounds. I have successfully maintained my ideal weight for more than five years. I will never go back to my old food choices. I made this decision because of the dramatic health benefits I realized when I changed my eating habits. I am healthier than I have been in years. The lifestyle change has made it easy to maintain the weight loss. I have seemingly endless amounts of energy, with no "low" spots during the day. An added bonus for me is that a bowel disease (called colitis) that I have battled for over 30 years has disappeared. I have not experienced any of the debilitating symptoms that I used to suffer since starting my low-carbohydrate approach to eating.

I made the decision to continue a low-carbohydrate lifestyle in order to maintain an optimum level of health and energy as well as an optimum weight. Once this decision was made, I determined I needed more variety and flavor in my diet. I have been interested in cooking and baking all my life, having learned the basics at a very early age from my mother. I have taken many culinary courses over the years and have picked up pointers from family and friends along the way.

When I decided to search out new and interesting recipes that met the low-carbohydrate standard, I was disappointed. When I reviewed what was available, I was not happy with the recipes, particularly the desserts. I still feel that dinner is not complete without dessert. I am content to have sugar-free Jell-O on some nights — but not every night — to adhere to a low-carbohydrate regime.

As part of my research, I went to the Internet, where a search resulted in no matches. That has changed: today there are many more options available for low-carb dieters. At the time that I was searching, I lamented the lack of resources and set about to create my own low-carbohydrate recipes. This became a fulfilling creative outlet as I developed new recipes and thought about how to modify some old standards to adhere to a low-carbohydrate approach.

One of my family members suggested I consider putting my recipes together; this cookbook is the result. I am thrilled to publish the third edition of *All New Easy Low-Carb Cooking* with many new and innovative recipes. Thanks to my family and friends who have contributed and to the many readers who have sent online submissions to our Recipe of the Month contest.

I have attempted to make the directions easy to follow and have tried to ensure that the ingredients are common to most kitchens. A few specialty ingredients that you may not recognize are described in the section titled "Low-Carb Cooking Tips." Some of these are necessary to provide the "glue" in certain recipes for muffins and cookies to avoid white wheat flour (which has gluten).

Because low-carbohydrate cooking and low-carbohydrate living may be new to some readers, I have included tips to guide you and ways to adjust your own favorite recipes.

In food preparation, we generally derive flavor from using either sugar or fat. Because low-carbohydrate diets limit the amount of sugar, much of the flavor comes from fats like cream and butter. These ingredients have been limited to allow you to maintain what I believe is a healthy balance of nutrients. You will note an increased use of the good fats, like extra virgin olive oil, and the essential fatty acids found in nuts. I have also used spices and fresh herbs to enhance the flavor and presentation of many dishes.

For every recipe in this cookbook, you will find nutritional information provided on a per serving basis. Some low-carbohydrate cookbooks provide the number of grams of carbohydrate for each serving without including the calorie or fat content. While I don't count calories, I do like to be able to balance my intake. If I have one menu item that is highly caloric, the other items on the menu will be less so to balance my daily intake. All nutritional information was calculated using the NutriBase IV Clinical Edition software from Cybersoft. Every effort has been made to ensure the accuracy of the nutritional information. In this edition all recipes mention the fiber content and the net carb content of the recipe. It is important for a healthy and balanced diet to ensure that you are ingesting sufficient fiber.

If you want to lose weight, I recommend that you visit your family doctor to make sure a low-carbohydrate approach to eating is appropriate for you. It is not my intention to convince readers that low-carbohydrate eating is the way to go, but rather to provide tools for those who have made the decision already.

Slow Carb for Life, coauthored with my physician husband, Harv Haakonson, was written to provide readers with a better understanding of the low-carb lifestyle. This book also provides menu planning for weight loss, maintenance, and entertaining using recipes from this cookbook. We have also written a section for adolescents and individuals who have special dietary needs, whether they are diabetic, vegetarian, or allergic to certain foods and include suggestions for eating out in restaurants or at friends' homes, feeding the rest of the family, and shopping. In addition, readers will find reviews of other low-carb diets, a personal Food Diary, and a 40-page Carbohydrate Counter. When we calculate net carb content, the only thing we deduct is the fiber contained in the recipe; we do not deduct the sugar substitute, and we do not use sugar alcohols in our recipes.

Readers often tell us our books are the ultimate guides to everyday low-carb living; I hope that you will feel the same and will enjoy experimenting with these recipes. I would be delighted to hear from you if you have a recipe you would like to see in future editions or if you have any questions. Contact me at www.slowcarbforlife.com.

Low-Carb Cooking Tips

Preparation

As with any other kind of cooking, it is best to be prepared when you are trying a new recipe. Read through the recipe before starting to ensure that you have all the ingredients on hand as well as the proper tools and equipment. I also like to make sure that my kitchen is clean and uncluttered before beginning.

Organization

It is easy to follow even a complicated recipe (there aren't many in this cookbook) by preparing the necessary ingredients before starting to cook. I measure and prepare all ingredients and put them in small dishes or containers so that they are at my fingertips when the recipe calls for them.

Herbs

I love to grow fresh herbs in pots just outside my kitchen. It doesn't take a lot of space or time, and it makes a wonderful difference in the taste, smell, and appearance of most dishes. It is somehow very satisfying to go out and snip a few herbs as I get ready to prepare a meal. I find that there is something relaxing and soothing about working with fragrant herbs. The ones that I always grow are flat leaf parsley and regular parsley, mint, thyme, lemon thyme, rosemary, dill, and chives. If you are unable or not inclined to grow fresh herbs, most markets and grocery stores sell them in the fresh produce section.

You will notice that I use a mix of dried herbs called Fine Herbs (or sometimes found with the French spelling of Fines Herbes) associated with French cuisine. Some mixes are better than others so I have included my own recipe. A store bought blend called Herbes de Provence is slightly different but also delicious.

Presentation

The presentation of a dish is important. I have included a number of simple ideas in the recipes: adding a sprig of mint or dill or using edible flowers (nasturtium or pansy) to garnish a salad or dessert, or using two cooked vegetables with different colors to make the plate look fuller. Attention to presentation will enhance the look of a dish and delight the senses.

Imagination

Once you become comfortable with low-carb cooking, you can begin to experiment to suit your own tastes. Change the herbs in a sauce or substitute a different vegetable in a salad or soup. A bit of imagination goes a long way. Keep in mind which ingredients you want to avoid. It is not as easy to experiment with baking, which is a bit like chemistry, where all the ingredients must be exact to achieve the desired results.

Equipment

It is easiest to prepare tasty meals if you have the right equipment. Tools don't have to be top of the line, but they must get the job done. One small piece of equipment that I recommend is a "rasp" or "zester" to get the zest from citrus fruits. You will also want to have a blender or food processor to make many of the soups and some of the muffins and cookies in the cookbook. I like to use an "immersion" blender for soups and veggies so you don't have to worry about putting the ingredients into one container to blend or purée and then transfer them to another one for continued heating or cooking.

Sugar Substitutes

There are many sugar substitutes available on the market; I prefer Splenda. This low-carb sweetener does not change flavor or texture when baking, does not contain aspartame, and it carries no known health risk. It is derived from sugar and is easy to use and widely available. I generally buy both the small packets and the granular form. The Splenda in packets is a concentrated form, equivalent to two teaspoons of sugar. It can also be purchased in granular form, which requires you to measure the amount needed. The granular form is not concentrated and may be used in equivalent measure to sugar. If you are following recipes in this cookbook and can only find the granular form, use two teaspoons for every packet in the recipe.

Some readers are interested in using stevia as a sugar substitute. Stevia is a natural product that provides sweetening, but I find it very difficult to work with for two reasons: it has a slight licorice taste that I find can overpower the other flavors in a dessert; and converting recipes or finding the correct amount to use can be a difficult task due to its potentcy.

A Word about Fats

Some of the recipes contain more fat than you may be used to to provide flavor and a feeling of satiation. Fats are essential for cell development and aid in the digestion of certain nutrients. The most important consideration when eating fat is to ensure it is one of the "good" fats like olive oil. You will not find margarine, with its hydrogenated ("bad") fats, anywhere in this cookbook. In addition, the fat content in many of the chicken, fish, and meat recipes comes from olive oil used in a marinade. While the olive oil must be included in the nutrition calculation, it is important to note that much of it stays behind in the dish when the food is cooked. This means the fat grams in the nutrition box will be slightly elevated compared to actual consumption.

Specialty Low-Carb Ingredients

Flax seed meal

This is a wonderful product that I discovered when developing low-carb muffins. It has many benefits that make it an appropriate ingredient in any balanced diet. Flax seed meal is a grain product that is very high in fiber and has omega-3 fatty acids (the good fats that we need for cell development). Flax seed meal has a wonderful nutty flavor and a dark rich color and texture to add to muffins, cookies, and breads. You can find flax seed meal in regular grocery stores (near the flours usually) or in health food stores. You can also purchase the flax as seeds and grind your own in a blender or coffee grinder. Even though it is a grain, flax seed or flax seed meal needs to be stored in the fridge.

Ground almonds

This ingredient is also known as almond meal, finely ground almonds that can be used as a flour substitute in many dishes. It has a very high fiber content, so the net carb is very low. It will not bind the way that flour does, so some additional ingredients are necessary when baking with almond meal.

Lindt chocolate

I often use this Swiss chocolate in baking because of its relatively low carbohydrate content compared with many other available chocolates. I particularly like the 70% cocoa, extra fine, rich dark chocolate for chocolate desserts. I also use the white chocolate in some recipes, but I never use the milk chocolate since it has too high a carb content. This chocolate comes in large bars (100 g each) and can be found in many grocery stores either in the baking section or in the candy section. I also find it in drugstores and in The Bay in Canada or Cost Plus stores in the United States.

Protein powders

These powders come in a variety of flavors and are very high in protein and low in carbs (be careful to purchase the low-carb protein powders). The protein may be whey based or soy based. You may need to go to a specialty health food or low-carb store to find them. They do tend to dry out a recipe, but they provide extra protein that makes the muffin satisfying.

Special flours

I use a number of different flours in this cookbook to minimize the use of white flour, which is a high-glycemic, high-carbohydrate ingredient. The substitutes that I use include soy flour, oat flour, and vital wheat gluten flour. All of these flours are available in regular grocery stores and in health food stores and are lower in carbs and higher in protein content than regular white flour. Experiment if you are adjusting your own recipes to see what works.

Xanthan gum

You need to go to a health food store to purchase this product. It is an essential ingredient in low-carb cooking if you want to bake cookies or thicken sauces. Xanthan gum is a fine white powder, much like cornstarch in consistency. You only need to purchase a small amount since it is very potent. This ingredient acts as the glue for other ingredients when you are baking without the gluten in wheat flour. It is also a great thickener for sauces.

Adjusting Your Family Favorites

If you want to experiment with adjusting favorite recipes your family doesn't want to give up, try to eliminate or drastically reduce any flour in the recipe. Other ingredients to keep to a minimum are cornstarch or other thickeners, rice, potato, and bread, including croutons and bread crumbs. In some cases, you can substitute ingredients to help make up for the lack of flour. For example, using light or heavy cream in a sauce rather than milk will allow you to reduce the need for flour. Sometimes you can add an egg or some cheese to make up for bread in a recipe. I welcome your recipe ideas at www.slowcarbforlife.com.

BREAKFAST FOODS

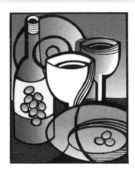

Baked Grapefruit

1 medium pink grapefruit
¼ teaspoon cinnamon
2 packets Splenda

- Preheat oven to 350°.
- Cut the grapefruit in half, and cut the sections with a grapefruit knife. Blend together the Splenda and cinnamon. Sprinkle the grapefruit halves with the spices.
- Place in a baking dish and bake for 20–25 minutes.
- Serve warm.

Makes 2 servings.

NOTE: This is a really exotic and delicious alternative to cold grapefruit. I always cut a small slice off each end to make a flat surface so that it sits better in the pan.

Nutrition Information per Serving

Calories	45.71
Protein	0.82 g
Carbs	11.57 g
Fat	0.14 g
Fiber	1.56 g
Net carb	10.01 g

Breakfast Pie

1 teaspoon butter
¼ cup heavy cream
1 cup canned pumpkin (not the pie filling)
½ teaspoon Dijon mustard
¼ teaspoon paprika
½ teaspoon fresh ground pepper
6 eggs

- Preheat oven to 375°.
- Whisk eggs with cream and spices. Add Dijon mustard to pumpkin and blend into egg mixture with a fork.
- Bake in a buttered 9″ glass pie plate until browned, about 25–30 minutes. *Makes 6 servings.*

NOTE: This is quite an unusual but tasty breakfast dish that can be reheated for lunch or dinner.

Nutrition Information per Serving

Calories	134.02
Protein	7.91 g
Carbs	4.70 g
Fat	9.26 g
Fiber	0.02 g
Net carb	4.68 g

Easy Cheesy Quiche

6 eggs
½ cup light cream (half & half)
½ cup heavy cream
1 cup freshly shredded cheddar cheese
½ teaspoon fresh ground pepper
¼ teaspoon salt
½ tablespoon fresh chopped parsley

- Preheat oven to 375°.
- Whisk eggs, both creams, and salt & pepper. Add the shredded cheese and blend gently with a fork.
- Pour into a buttered quiche dish or a 9″ pie plate.
- Bake for 25–30 minutes until lightly browned.

Makes 6 servings.

NOTE: This is also good reheated the following day for lunch or dinner.

Nutrition Information per Serving

Calories	396.25
Protein	20.26 g
Carbs	4.27 g
Fat	32.95 g
Fiber	0.04 g
Net carb	4.23 g

Eggs Benedict

4 eggs
¼″ thick ham steak or small round ham
1 tablespoon olive oil
1 beefsteak tomato
½ cup Hollandaise Sauce (see recipe)
dash of paprika

- Heat olive oil in a frying pan over medium heat.
- Cut small ham into ¼″ slices, or cut ham steak into 3″ squares.
- Put ham in frying pan and brown on both sides. Remove from pan and place in a warm oven (approximately 250°).
- Cut tomato into ¼″ slices and cook in frying pan for just a minute or so on each side. Remove to warm oven.
- Poach 4 eggs for approximately 4 minutes. Eggs may be poached in the microwave, which will shorten cooking time, or in an electric poacher.
- To poach eggs in the frying pan, fill it with 1″ of water, crack the egg into a small dish or ramekin, and gently pour the egg into the boiling water to retain its shape. You may need to spoon the boiling water over the top of the yolk to ensure that it is properly cooked.
- To assemble the dish, place warm ham on the plate, then layer with cooked tomato and egg. Cover with warm Hollandaise Sauce. Sprinkle with paprika.

Makes 2 servings.

NOTE: This is a really delicious alternative to the other eggs Benedict. The most difficult part is the timing of the sauce and the eggs. An egg poacher goes a long way in simplifying the process.

Nutrition Information per Serving

Calories	293.97
Protein	23.86 g
Carbs	4.99 g
Fat	19.10 g
Fiber	0.33 g
Net carb	4.66 g

Granola

....

1 cup All Bran Extra Fiber

1 cup rolled oats (not the instant variety)

½ cup soy nuts

½ cup slivered almonds

½ cup sunflower seeds

1 teaspoon cinnamon

¼ cup sugar-free syrup

- Preheat oven to 350°.
- Mix all ingredients together in a large bowl. Pour syrup over ingredients and stir to coat. Use just enough of any sugar-free syrup to allow mixture to bind. Place in a single layer on a cookie sheet covered with parchment paper.
- Bake for 25–30 minutes, stirring twice during the baking.
- Let cool completely and store in an airtight container.

Makes 4 cups of granola and 8 servings of ½cup each.

NOTE: This might seem like a lot of trouble, but it is a very tasty granola, and you can be sure of all the contents and the carb count. Make your own variety by adding a few raisins, some flax seed meal, or other nuts.

Nutrition Information per Serving

Calories	174.39
Protein	11.35 g
Carbs	18.29 g
Fat	9.93 g
Fiber	10.22 g
Net carb	8.07 g

Hash Browns

2 tablespoons olive oil
2 cups cabbage, cut into 1″ pieces
¼ cup minced onion
1 cup pork rinds, roughly chopped
salt & ground pepper to taste

• Heat the olive oil over medium heat and add cabbage and onion. Sauté until tender, approximately 6–10 minutes.
• Add salt & pepper. Add the chopped pork rinds and continue to cook for 2 or 3 more minutes until everything is heated through and blended.
Makes 2 servings of approximately 1 cup each.

NOTE: This recipe calls for 1 cup of pork rinds before chopping or approximately 1/2 cup when chopped. The pork rinds add a really nice bacon flavor and some crispness to the dish. This is a great substitute for hash browns with breakfast.

Nutrition Information per Serving

Calories	166.20
Protein	1.94 g
Carbs	9.73 g
Fat	14.70 g
Fiber	3.87 g
Net carb	5.86 g

Mushroom & Cheese Omelet

2 eggs
2 teaspoons butter
1 tablespoon water
½ cup sliced fresh mushrooms
¼ cup shredded cheddar cheese
fresh ground pepper & salt to taste

• Melt 1 teaspoon of butter in small frying pan and sauté mushrooms until soft. Set aside but keep warm.
• Add water to eggs and beat with whisk until smooth. Add ground pepper & salt to taste.
• Wipe out frying pan and add second teaspoon of butter and melt over medium heat. Rotate pan to ensure that butter coats bottom and sides evenly.
• Pour eggs into pan, rotating to ensure that the bottom is evenly distributed. As egg sets around the edges, lift with a spatula to allow uncooked egg to run under edges. When egg is mostly cooked, add mushrooms and cheese. Slip spatula under one side and gently fold omelet over to form a half moon, and let sit for another minute to melt cheese. Using spatula, slide omelet onto serving dish. *Makes 1 serving.*

VARIATIONS: The following fillings can be used to vary the omelet.
Peppers: sautéed chopped red and green peppers.
Fine herbs: freshly chopped parsley, chives, and thyme.
Western: ham, green pepper, and onion.
Vegetable: sautéed green onion, zucchini, and cheese, or any vegetable you like.

NOTE: This omelet can be made with egg beaters or just egg whites if preferred.

Nutrition Information per Serving	
Calories	350.47
Protein	22.13 g
Carbs	3.80 g
Fat	27.16 g
Fiber	0.42 g
Net carb	3.38 g

Mushroom & Spinach Frittata

1 teaspoon butter
1 small onion, halved & sliced
1 cup fresh sliced mushrooms
1 cup cooked fresh spinach,
  chopped
1 tablespoon fresh chopped
  parsley
⅛ teaspoon cayenne

8 eggs, beaten
¼ cup light cream (half & half)
½ teaspoon Dijon mustard
½ teaspoon salt
1 teaspoon fresh ground pepper
½ cup shredded cheddar cheese
1 tablespoon toasted pine nuts

• Preheat oven to 375°.
• Lightly grease a 9″ glass pie plate.
• Melt butter in a nonstick frying pan over medium heat. Add onion and mushrooms and sauté until soft, approximately 5 minutes. Remove from heat and add the cooked chopped spinach, parsley, and cayenne.
• In a bowl, whisk the eggs, half & half, mustard, salt, and pepper. Stir in the vegetable mixture and cheese. Pour mixture into the pie plate and sprinkle with pine nuts.
• Bake for 25–30 minutes until top is nicely browned. Remove from oven and serve immediately.
Makes 6 servings.

NOTE: This is a gorgeous-looking browned egg and vegetable dish reminiscent of a quiche without the pastry. It can be served for either breakfast or lunch.

Nutrition Information per Serving	
Calories	179.76
Protein	12.80 g
Carbs	3.59 g
Fat	12.41 g
Fiber	0.42 g
Net carb	3.17 g

Strawberry Smoothie

2 scoops (about 3 tablespoons) strawberry-flavored protein powder
½ cup frozen strawberries
¾ cup water

- Put all ingredients in a blender and process until smooth.

NOTE: If you want to cut your carb count, reduce the amount of frozen berries. Doing so will make the shake a little thinner in texture. You can also add just a tablespoon of heavy cream to add to the creamy texture of your shake.

Nutrition Information per Serving	
Calories	86.08
Protein	10.32 g
Carbs	8.80 g
Fat	1.08 g
Fiber	2.56 g
Net carb	6.24 g

Sausage Pie

1 sausage (4–5 ounces)

6 large eggs

4 green onions, sliced

1 zucchini, quartered and cut into small pieces

½ red or green bell pepper, diced

½ cup light cream

1 cup shredded sharp cheddar cheese

1 teaspoon salt

½ teaspoon black pepper

- If the sausage has a casing, remove and discard it. Cut the sausage into bite-sized pieces. Cook the sausage in a large skillet until it crumbles.
- Preheat oven to 325°.
- Add green onion, zucchini, and bell pepper and sauté until soft, about 5 minutes. Drain excess fat from dish.
- Whisk egg and light cream until blended. Add salt & pepper.
- In a lightly greased 9″ pie plate, place sausage and vegetable mixture, layer with cheese, and then pour egg mixture over all.
- At this point, you may cover and place the pie in the fridge overnight or for a few hours, or you may put the pie directly into the hot oven.
- Bake uncovered at 325° for 45–50 minutes if baking immediately, until edges are brown and egg is set. If taking out of the fridge, bake for 60 minutes.

Makes 6 servings.

NOTE: This is a great dish for breakfast, brunch, or lunch. Use any type of sausage, depending on your preferences.

Nutrition Information per Serving	
Calories	303.52
Protein	16.01 g
Carbs	5.47 g
Fat	23.83 g
Fiber	0.72 g
Net carb	4.75 g

Waffles

1 cup soy flour
1 tablespoon baking powder
3 packets Splenda
1 teaspoon salt
¼ cup heavy cream
¾ cup water
3 eggs
1 teaspoon vanilla

- Mix dry ingredients together in a bowl.
- Beat eggs until foamy in a separate bowl. Add remaining ingredients to eggs.
- Combine both wet and dry ingredients and mix well. This will make a very thick batter.
- Cook in a waffle iron, according to instructions.
- Serve with whipped cream, some jam (no sugar added), or fresh or frozen fruit.

Makes 6 waffles.

NOTE: The nutrition information was calculated for the waffles only. Be sure to calculate the additional carbs for whichever topping you choose.

TIP: If you do not have a waffle iron, you can make pancakes.

Thanks to Lynn Beach from Weyburn, Saskatchewan, for this recipe.

Nutrition Information per Serving

Calories	154.56
Protein	9.70 g
Carbs	8.37 g
Fat	9.50 g
Fiber	2.67 g
Net carb	5.70 g

BREADS & MUFFINS

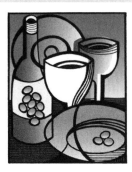

Basic Bread

1½ cups warm water
½ tablespoon active dry yeast
2 cups vital wheat gluten flour
1 egg
1 tablespoon olive oil
¼ teaspoon salt
1 tablespoon Splenda

• Add all ingredients in the order listed to your bread machine.
• Bake bread on the whole wheat setting on your machine. Set the crust setting to light if this option is available.
Makes approximately 10–12 slices.

NOTE: This bread can be made only with a bread machine because of the heavy elastic nature of the vital wheat gluten flour. This flour is high in protein and low in carbohydrates and can be found in the baking section of most grocery stores. Look for Bob's Red Mill brand, which is a popular variety of alternative flours and other baking ingredients. The recipe makes one decent-sized loaf.

Nutrition Information per Serving	
Calories	116.59
Protein	19.18 g
Carbs	5.13 g
Fat	17.31 g
Fiber	0.04 g
Net carb	5.09 g

NOTE: Nutrition information is based on a single slice, using 10 slices total for the loaf of bread.

Thanks to Joseph Gallacher of Victoria, British Columbia, for this tasty recipe, which inspired me to experiment with other varieties of low-carb breads.

Coconut Zucchini Muffins

½ cup ground almonds
¼ cup each ground sesame &
    sunflower seeds
½ cup flax seed meal
¼ cup soy flour
2 packets Splenda
½ teaspoon baking soda
½ teaspoon baking powder
½ teaspoon xanthan gum

¼ teaspoon salt
¼ cup sweetened coconut
1 egg, beaten
2 tablespoons olive oil
½ teaspoon coconut extract
¼ cup water
1 cup finely shredded zucchini
    (1 medium)

- Preheat oven to 375°.
- The nuts and seeds may be ground in a food processor.
- Mix all dry ingredients together. Mix wet ingredients in a separate bowl.
- Add wet ingredients to dry and stir to blend. Pour into muffin tins that have been lined with paper muffin cups.
- Bake for 25 minutes, until brown around the edges.

Makes 8 muffins.

VARIATION: You can substitute pumpkin seeds for the sesame seeds.

Many thanks to my sister Stephanie Tompkins for developing this recipe.

Nutrition Information per Serving

Calories	162.08
Protein	6.01 g
Carbs	5.43 g
Fat	13.85 g
Fiber	0.53 g
Net carb	4.90 g

Flax & Oat Bread

1¼ cups warm water
1 tablespoon olive oil
¼ teaspoon salt
1 egg
1 cup vital wheat gluten flour
½ cup flax seed meal
¼ cup oat flour
¼ cup soy flour
1 tablespoon Splenda
½ tablespoon active dry yeast

- Add all ingredients in the order listed to your bread machine.
- Bake bread on the whole wheat setting on your machine. Set the crust setting to light if this option is available.

Makes approximately 10–12 slices.

NOTE: This bread can only be made with a bread machine because of the heavy elastic nature of the vital wheat gluten flour. This flour is high in protein and low in carbohydrates and can be found in the baking section of most grocery stores. Look for Bob's Red Mill brand, which is a popular variety of alternative flours and other baking ingredients. The recipe makes one good-sized loaf.

Nutrition Information per Serving	
Calories	74.80
Protein	9.50 g
Carbs	4.44 g
Fat	2.31 g
Fiber	0.69 g
Net carb	3.75 g

NOTE: Nutrition information is based on a single slice, using 10 slices total for the loaf of bread.

Flax & Oat Muffins

....

1 cup oat flour

½ cup soy flour

½ cup flax seed meal

½ teaspoon salt

2 teaspoons baking powder

⅔ cup light cream (half & half)

2 tablespoons olive oil

2 eggs

- Preheat oven to 425°.
- Mix all dry ingredients in a bowl.
- Whisk together eggs; then continue whisking as you add the other wet ingredients.
- Make a well in the dry ingredients, pour in the egg mixture, and mix thoroughly with a wooden spoon.
- Pour into a nonstick muffin pan.
- Bake for 15–18 minutes or until browned on top.

Makes 10 muffins.

VARIATION: These can be made into biscuits by dropping them on a nonstick cookie sheet and baking. For variety, try adding some bacon bits, chopped green onion, or dry herbs to the dough.

Nutrition Information per Serving

Calories	152.21
Protein	7.89 g
Carbs	11.60 g
Fat	8.90 g
Fiber	3.36 g
Net carb	8.24 g

Lemon Carrot Muffins

½ cup ground almonds
(or walnuts)
¼ cup each ground sesame and
sunflower seeds
½ cup flax seed meal
¼ cup soy flour
2 packets Splenda
½ teaspoon baking soda
½ teaspoon baking powder

½ teaspoon xanthan gum
¼ teaspoon salt
zest and juice of half a lemon
¼ cup raisins
1 egg, beaten
2 tablespoons olive oil
¼ cup plus 2 tablespoons water
1½ cups finely shredded carrot (2
medium)

• Preheat oven to 375°.
• The nuts and seeds may be ground in a food processor. The lemon zest needs
to be very fine.
• Mix all dry ingredients together. Mix wet ingredients in a separate bowl.
• Add wet ingredients to dry and stir to blend. Pour into muffin tins that have
been lined with paper muffin cups.
• Bake for 25 minutes, until brown around the edges.
Makes 8 muffins.

VARIATION: You may use orange juice and zest instead of lemon, but this will increase your carb count slightly. Substitute pumpkin seeds in place of sesame seeds.

Thanks again to my sister Stephanie Tompkins for developing this recipe.

**Nutrition Information
per Serving**

Calories	169.77
Protein	6.12 g
Carbs	10.37 g
Fat	12.29 g
Fiber	1.40 g
Net carb	8.97 g

Magic Muffins

2 eggs, separated
5 tablespoons light olive oil
1 teaspoon vanilla
1 teaspoon baking powder
1 teaspoon cinnamon
¼ teaspoon nutmeg
2 packets Splenda
½ cup ground almonds
½ cup ground pecans
   (or walnuts)

1 cup flax seed meal
¼ cup whey (or soy) protein
   powder
1 cup finely shredded zucchini
1 cup finely shredded cabbage
½ cup finely shredded carrot
½ cup finely chopped
   cauliflower

- Preheat oven to 375°.
- Line a 12-medium-sized muffin tin with paper liners.
- Beat room temperature egg whites with a pinch of salt until stiff peaks form. Set aside.
- Finely shred and chop the vegetables, either by hand or in a food processor. Chop the nuts, or use a food processor on pulse for about 10 seconds. You do not want to pulverize the nuts, but they need to be very small. Combine the nuts and vegetables and blend well.
- Whisk together the egg yolks, olive oil, vanilla, cinnamon, nutmeg, Splenda, and baking powder until well mixed. Add the flax seed meal and the protein powder. This becomes a fairly dense mixture.
- Add the nuts and vegetables to the flax mixture and mix well. Fold in the egg white until blended.

continued

• Spoon the mixture into the lined muffin molds. Bake for 30–40 minutes, until nicely browned on top.

Makes 12 muffins.

VARIATION: You can vary the nuts to alter the flavor of these muffins. You may also substitute different vegetables, using yellow summer squash or broccoli, if desired. For the protein powder, you can use a vanilla or unflavored protein shake mix if you have one in your cupboard, or purchase one at the health food store. My friend Annette Wall suggested substituting savory seasonings for the cinnamon to make a savory muffin to have with soup.

Nutrition Information per Serving	
Calories	194.02
Protein	5.74 g
Carbs	7.60 g
Fat	16.75 g
Fiber	5.08 g
Net carb	2.52 g

Thanks to Valerie Caspersen of Victoria, British Columbia, who gave me the idea for these great muffins.

Oat Bran Bread

1 ¾ cups vital wheat gluten flour

2 tablespoons wheat bran

2 tablespoons oat bran

¼ cup flax seed meal

½ cup soy flour

1 tablespoon dry active yeast

1 tablespoon olive oil

½ cup water

2 eggs

½ teaspoon salt

• The water and eggs combined must equal 1 cup in total volume.
• Put all liquid ingredients in the bottom of a bread machine and add the salt.
• Mix all dry ingredients except the yeast in a large bowl and stir to blend. Put the dry ingredients into the bread maker. Make a well in the top and add the yeast.
• Set the bread maker to whole wheat setting, with a light crust if that is an option.
• This is a large and heavy loaf, and you will need a bread maker capable of a 2-pound loaf. It will give your machine a workout.
This loaf should provide 14 slices of bread.

NOTE: The nutrition information is calculated per slice.

Thanks to Bendt Caspersen of Victoria, British Columbia, for this recipe. Bendt notes that he does not have a bread maker but uses his Kitchen Aid mixer to mix the dough, lets the dough rise twice, and then bakes at 350° for an hour.

Nutrition Information per Serving

Calories	108.00
Protein	15.66 g
Carbs	6.41 g
Fat	2.84 g
Fiber	1.13 g
Net carb	5.28 g

Oatmeal Flax Muffins

¾ cup vanilla whey protein
   powder

½ cup rolled oats

½ cup flax seed meal

2 tablespoons egg white powder

1 teaspoon baking powder

1 teaspoon cinnamon

½ teaspoon nutmeg

¼ teaspoon ground cloves

⅔ cup Splenda

⅛ teaspoon salt

½ cup canned pumpkin

1 tablespoon orange zest

¼ cup fresh orange juice

¼ cup water

¼ cup heavy cream

¼ cup chopped walnuts

3 large eggs

3 tablespoons olive oil

- Preheat oven to 350°.
- Spray a muffin pan with a nonstick agent and set aside.
- Mix all dry ingredients in a large bowl. The walnuts can be added after the other ingredients have been well blended.
- Whisk the eggs with the olive oil and then add the other wet ingredients, including the canned pumpkin, orange zest, and juice. It is easiest to add the pumpkin using a fork to blend.
- Make a well in the dry ingredients and pour the wet ingredients into the well. Blend well with a wooden spoon.
- Pour into the prepared muffin pan and bake for approximately 25–30 minutes, until edges are browned.

Makes 12 muffins.

VARIATION: You can substitute a 1/4 cup of raisins for the walnuts, although they will increase the carb content slightly.

Nutrition Information per Serving	
Calories	139.71
Protein	5.80 g
Carbs	6.50 g
Fat	10.57 g
Fiber	2.34 g
Net carb	4.16 g

Oatmeal Pumpkin Muffins

1½ cups canned pumpkin, not the pie filling

1 teaspoon baking powder

1 teaspoon cinnamon

½ teaspoon nutmeg

¼ teaspoon ginger

¼ cup flax seed meal

½ cup vanilla whey protein

¼ cup oatmeal

9 packets Splenda

2 tablespoons egg white powder

¼ cup walnuts

¼ cup heavy cream

3 eggs

3 tablespoons olive oil

- Preheat oven to 375°.
- Spray muffin pan with a nonstick agent.
- Mix all dry ingredients in a bowl.
- In a separate bowl, whisk together eggs and oil. Add cream while continuing to whisk.
- Make a well in the dry ingredients. Add the wet ingredients and stir until well blended.
- Pour into prepared muffin pan and bake for 25–30 minutes, until brown at the edges.
Makes 12 muffins.

NOTE: Powdered egg white can be found in most health food stores.

Nutrition Information per Serving	
Calories	133.28
Protein	7.27 g
Carbs	5.86 g
Fat	9.69 g
Fiber	1.27 g
Net carb	4.59 g

Orange Cranberry Muffins

¾ cup vanilla whey protein powder

½ cup soy flour

½ cup flax seed meal

2 tablespoons egg white powder

1 teaspoon baking powder

¼ teaspoon ground ginger

½ teaspoon nutmeg

¼ teaspoon ground cloves

¼ cup Splenda

1 cup fresh cranberries, roughly chopped

zest & juice of a fresh orange

¼ cup water

¼ cup heavy cream

3 large eggs

3 tablespoons olive oil

- Preheat oven to 350°.
- Spray a muffin pan with a nonstick agent and set aside.
- Mix all dry ingredients in a large bowl.
- Whisk the eggs with the olive oil and then add the other wet ingredients, including the cranberries, orange zest, and juice.
- Make a well in the dry ingredients and pour the wet ingredients into the well. Blend well with a wooden spoon.
- Pour into the prepared muffin pan and bake for approximately 25–30 minutes, until edges are browned.

Makes 12 muffins.

VARIATION: You can substitute a 1/4 cup of dried cranberries for the fresh, although they will increase the carb content slightly. These muffins have a surprisingly pleasant tart note thanks to the cranberries. You will lose the tartness if you use the dried cranberries since they are much sweeter.

Nutrition Information per Serving

Calories	151.72
Protein	10.94 g
Carbs	7.53 g
Fat	9.18 g
Fiber	2.61 g
Net carb	4.92 g

Raisin Flax Muffins

3 eggs
3 tablespoons butter
¼ cup water
3 tablespoons extra virgin olive oil
½ cup vanilla whey protein powder
2 tablespoons soy flour
2 teaspoons baking powder
3 tablespoons flax seed meal
6 packets Splenda
¼ cup raisins

- Preheat oven to 350°.
- Separate eggs and beat egg whites until they form stiff peaks.
- In a medium bowl, beat egg yolks with butter and olive oil and water.
- In a separate bowl, mix whey protein, soy flour, flax seed meal, raisins, Splenda, and baking powder.
- Beat dry mixture into egg yolk combination. Gently fold egg whites into batter and pour into a buttered nonstick muffin pan.
- Bake for 25–30 minutes, until inserted toothpick comes out clean.
Makes 8 muffins.

NOTE: If you want to reduce the carb content, reduce the amount of raisins.

Nutrition Information per Serving

Calories	178.68
Protein	7.40 g
Carbs	7.98 g
Fat	13.33 g
Fiber	1.85 g
Net carb	6.13 g

Walnut Flax Muffins

3 eggs, separated
3 tablespoons butter, melted
3 tablespoons light olive oil
½ cup vanilla whey protein powder
2 tablespoons soy flour
3 tablespoons flax seed meal
¼ cup walnuts, chopped
¼ cup water
½ teaspoon ground cinnamon
6 packets Splenda
2 teaspoons baking powder

- Separate eggs and beat egg whites until they form stiff peaks.
- In a medium bowl, whisk egg yolks with butter, olive oil, and water.
- In a separate bowl, sift whey protein, soy flour, cinnamon, Splenda, and baking powder. Add flax seed meal and walnuts and mix with a large wooden spoon.
- Blend dry mixture into egg yolk combination.
- Gently fold egg whites into batter and pour into a nonstick muffin pan that has been sprayed with a nonstick agent.
- Bake in a preheated oven at 350° for 25–30 minutes, until inserted toothpick comes out clean. The muffins will be golden brown on top with a slight sheen.

Makes 10 muffins.

Nutrition Information per Serving	
Calories	148.36
Protein	6.58 g
Carbs	3.78 g
Fat	12.37 g
Fiber	1.34 g
Net carb	2.44 g

Walnut Pumpkin Loaf

¾ cup vanilla whey protein
   powder
2 tablespoons egg white powder
1 tablespoon baking powder
1 teaspoon cinnamon
½ tablespoon ground cloves
½ teaspoon nutmeg
⅛ teaspoon mace
⅛ teaspoon ginger

⅔ cup Splenda
⅛ teaspoon salt
1½ cups canned pumpkin (not
   pie filling)
¼ cup heavy cream
¼ cup chopped walnuts
3 large eggs
3 tablespoons olive oil
2 tablespoons water

• Preheat oven to 375°.
• Spray a 9″ x 3″ x 5″ loaf pan with a nonstick agent and set aside.
• Mix all dry ingredients in a large bowl. The walnuts can be added after the
other ingredients have been well blended.
• Whisk the eggs with the olive oil and then add the other wet ingredients,
including the canned pumpkin. It is easiest to add the pumpkin using a fork to
blend.
• Make a well in the dry ingredients and pour the wet ingredients into the well.
Blend well with a wooden spoon.
• Pour into the prepared loaf pan and bake for
approximately 1 hour and 10 minutes. Test with
a toothpick.
• Let cool before cutting.
Makes approximately 12 slices.

NOTE: This is a wonderful midmorning or
afternoon snack with a cup of tea.

My thanks to Louise Armstrong for inspiring
this recipe.

Nutrition Information per Serving	
Calories	106.89
Protein	4.43 g
Carbs	4.53 g
Fat	8.28 g
Fiber	0.33 g
Net carb	4.20 g

Whole Wheat Flax Bread

1 cup and 2 tablespoons warm water
1 tablespoon olive oil
½ teaspoon salt
½ tablespoon dry active yeast
4 packets Splenda
1 cup vital wheat gluten flour
½ cup whole wheat flour
½ cup flax seed meal
½ cup wheat bran

• Place liquid ingredients in the bottom of a bread maker pan. Add the salt to the wet ingredients.
• Mix all dry ingredients, except the yeast, together in a bowl.
• Gently add the dry ingredients to the bread maker pan. Make a well in the top of the dry ingredients and add the yeast.
• Bake on the whole wheat setting, with a light crust if that is an option.
Makes a nice loaf with 12 slices of bread.

NOTE: This bread has a slightly higher carb count due to the whole wheat flour, but it is really delicious and worth the extra carbs once in a while. It is still well below any commercial breads in terms of carb content.

Nutrition Information per Serving

Calories	96.09
Protein	9.88 g
Carbs	9.15 g
Fat	3.87 g
Fiber	3.05 g
Net carb	6.10 g

APPETIZERS
& SNACKS

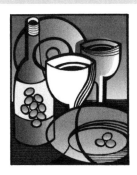

Avocado Dip

....

½ cup sour cream
½ cup mayonnaise
1 small ripe avocado
2 green onions, chopped
⅔ cup chopped fresh parsley
2 tablespoons fresh lemon juice
1 clove garlic, minced
1 tablespoon chopped fresh thyme

- Peel avocado and remove the pit. Cut into small pieces.
- Put all ingredients into a blender or food processor and process until smooth.
- Place dip in a small bowl, cover with plastic wrap, and refrigerate for 2–3 hours. Just before serving, garnish with some chopped fresh parsley.
- Serve with slices of cucumber, zucchini, or small crackers.

Makes approximately 2 cups.

NOTE: This dip is a beautiful green with dark flecks from the fresh herbs. It tastes wonderful and is so easy to make. The nutrition information is based on 50 servings.

Nutrition Information per Serving

Calories	28.22
Protein	0.13 g
Carbs	0.81 g
Fat	2.79 g
Fiber	0.35 g
Net carb	0.46 g

Cheese & Salmon Ball

6 ounces salmon, canned or
  fresh cooked
8 ounces cream cheese
¼ cup red onion, minced
½ teaspoon chili powder
4 ounces cheddar cheese,
  shredded

1 tablespoon sour cream
1 large egg, hard-boiled
¼ cup cashews
2 tablespoons chopped fresh
  parsley

• Mix all ingredients except the nuts and parsley. It is easiest to do this with a hand mixer, being careful not to purée the mixture.
• Divide the mixture into two equal parts. Place each batch into a small round bowl, press down, and cover with plastic wrap. Place in the fridge for 2–3 hours.
• Invert the mixture onto the plastic wrap and use hands to even out any irregularities in the ball. At this point, either one or both balls may be double-wrapped and frozen. You may add the nuts before freezing, but leave the parsley until just ready to serve as it does not freeze well.
• To finish, roughly chop nuts and parsley together. Place nut and parsley mixture on some wax paper and roll the cheese ball in the mixture, pressing lightly to ensure that the nuts and parsley adhere.
Makes 2 balls of approximately 25–30 servings each.

NOTE: I serve these with fresh vegetables: both carrot and celery sticks and cucumber and zucchini rounds. Nutrition information is calculated based on 50 servings of the cheese & salmon ball only.

Thanks to Joseph Gallacher of Victoria, British Columbia, for this delicious recipe.

Nutrition Information per Serving	
Calories	33.08
Protein	1.82 g
Carbs	0.53 g
Fat	2.67 g
Fiber	0.04 g
Net carb	0.49 g

Chocolate Nut Protein Bar

¼ cup soy protein powder

¼ cup unsalted peanuts

¼ cup pecans (or walnuts)

¼ cup almond slivers

¼ cup sunflower seeds

¼ cup pumpkin seeds

1 tablespoon oat flour

2 tablespoons unsweetened cocoa
   powder

6 packets Splenda

2 tablespoons whey protein powder

½ tablespoon xanthan gum

2–4 tablespoons water

1 teaspoon vanilla extract

2 tablespoons heavy cream

2 tablespoons olive oil

1 beaten egg

2 tablespoons peanut butter

2 tablespoons chocolate-flavored
   protein powder

• Preheat oven to 350°.
• Spray loaf pan with a nonstick agent.
• Put all dry ingredients in a food processor and blend well. (I leave a few pieces a bit bigger to provide texture and crunch.)
• Whisk egg and add olive oil, then water and cream. Finally, add peanut butter and vanilla to liquid and blend with whisk.
• Add dry ingredients to the wet and blend with a large spoon (use just enough water to allow you to blend the mixture). This will make a sticky and heavy batter.
• Place batter in loaf pan and spread evenly with the back of a spoon. Bake for 25 minutes, until golden brown at the edges.
Let cool.
Cut into 8 even bars.

NOTE: The flavor is somewhat dependent on the cocoa powder that you use. I use a rich dark cocoa powder. These freeze well.

Thanks to my sister Stephanie Tompkins, who did all the difficult preliminary work on these bars.

Nutrition Information per Serving	
Calories	222.91
Protein	9.56 g
Carbs	7.32 g
Fat	18.26 g
Fiber	0.89 g
Net carb	6.43 g

Citrus Protein Bar

¼ cup soy protein powder

1 teaspoon cinnamon

1 teaspoon nutmeg

¼ cup pecans (or walnuts)

¼ cup almond slivers

¼ cup sunflower seeds

¼ cup pumpkin seeds

¼ cup unsweetened coconut

4 packets Splenda

3 tablespoons whey protein powder

1 tablespoon xanthan gum

¼ cup water

zest of 1 lemon

2 tablespoons light cream

2 tablespoons olive oil

1 beaten egg

2 tablespoons no-sugar-added apricot jam

- Preheat oven to 350°.
- Spray loaf pan with a nonstick agent.
- Put all dry ingredients in a food processor and blend well. (I leave a few pieces a bit bigger to provide texture and crunch.)
- Whisk egg and add olive oil, then water and light cream. Finally, add jam and fine lemon zest to liquid and blend with whisk.
- Add dry ingredients to the wet and blend with a large spoon. This will make a sticky and heavy batter.
- Place batter in loaf pan and spread evenly with the back of a spoon. Bake for 25 minutes, until golden brown at the edges. Let cool.

Cut into 8 even bars.

VARIATION: Change the flavor with different jams. E.D. Smith makes a strawberry and a blackberry no-sugar-added jam that would be nice in these bars.

Thanks to my sister Stephanie Tompkins, who did all the difficult preliminary work on these bars.

Nutrition Information per Serving	
Calories	177.47
Protein	7.21 g
Carbs	5.44 g
Fat	14.94 g
Fiber	0.96 g
Net carb	4.48 g

Crab Dip

1 package (250 grams)
  Philadelphia Cream Cheese
1 can (120 grams) crab meat
1 cup mayonnaise

1 tablespoon Sambal Oelek (hot
  chili sauce)
½ cup finely shredded cheddar
  cheese

- Preheat oven to 350°.
- Cut Philadelphia cheese into chunks and place in an oven-proof dish (either 1.5- or 2-quart dish). Place a cover on the dish and heat the cheese in the oven for approximately 15 minutes.
- While the cheese is in the oven, mix the crab meat with the mayonnaise and the hot chili sauce until well blended.
- Remove the cheese from the oven and add the crab mixture. Mix well and scrape down the sides of the dish with a spatula.
- Replace the dish, still covered, in the oven for 20 minutes. Then remove from the oven and sprinkle the grated cheddar cheese on top and put back in the oven, uncovered, for 5–10 minutes, until the cheese is melted and the crab mixture is brown at the edges.
- Serve warm or cold with fresh veggies for dipping.

Makes approximately 48 servings of 2 teaspoons each.

VARIATION: Use shredded Swiss cheese. This will be a slightly more subtle taste addition, and the color will blend well with the crab. Another variation might be to add a little more of the hot chili sauce, depending on your taste buds. As it appears here, it has a nice little afterbite!

NOTE: You will probably find the Sambal Oelek, a hot chili sauce, in the Chinese-cooking section of your grocery store.

Nutrition Information per Serving	
Calories	50.33
Protein	1.29 g
Carbs	0.39 g
Fat	4.89 g
Fiber	0.00 g
Net carb	0.39 g

Thanks to Joanne Francis of Delta, British Columbia, for this delicious recipe.

Curried Crab

¾ cup chopped crab meat
½ cup finely chopped celery
½ cup real mayonnaise
2 tablespoons chopped green onion
1 tablespoon dried parsley
1 teaspoon curry powder
½ teaspoon dried mustard
⅛ teaspoon cayenne pepper
freshly ground pepper & salt, to taste
1 small English cucumber, sliced
1 teaspoon freshly minced parsley, to garnish

• Put all ingredients, except the cucumber, in medium bowl and mix well. The curried crab meat will keep well in the fridge for up to a full day.
• Place a small amount of crab meat on each cucumber slice. (You may also use small wheat crackers, although they will dramatically increase the carbohydrates.)
• Place on serving platter and garnish with freshly minced parsley.
Makes approximately 48 pieces.

Nutrition Information per Serving	
Calories	21.17
Protein	0.88 g
Carbs	0.13 g
Fat	1.90 g
Fiber	0.05 g
Net carb	0.08 g

Deviled Eggs with Chives

6 eggs
2 tablespoons sour cream
2 tablespoons mayonnaise
2 teaspoons fresh lemon juice
2 teaspoons chopped fresh chives
1 teaspoon Dijon mustard
pinch of paprika

• Place eggs in a saucepan with enough water to cover them. Bring water to a boil and cook for 10 minutes. Remove eggs from hot water and wash with cold water until eggs are cool. Refrigerate for 30 minutes to cool completely.
• Crack the eggshells all around and peel shells. Cut eggs in half lengthwise. Remove yolks carefully and place whites on serving dish.
• In a small bowl, crush yolks with a fork. Add all remaining ingredients except paprika and whisk until smooth.
• Spoon the yolk mixture into the hollow whites and swirl the tops. Sprinkle with a dash of paprika to add color.
Makes 12 servings.

Nutrition Information per Serving	
Calories	56.07
Protein	3.22 g
Carbs	0.58 g
Fat	4.53 g
Fiber	0.01 g
Net carb	0.57 g

Glazed Walnuts

3 cups walnuts
4 packets Splenda
1 teaspoon paprika
½ teaspoon cayenne
½ teaspoon nutmeg
¼ cup soy sauce
1 tablespoon butter

• Preheat oven to 250°.
• Melt butter and mix with soy sauce, Splenda, and spices. Place nuts in a large bowl and pour butter and spice mixture over nuts. Stir to coat.
• Line a cookie sheet with parchment paper. Arrange nuts in a single layer on cookie sheet. Use a rubber spatula to scrape bowl and pour any leftover sauce on the walnuts.
• Bake for approximately 30–35 minutes or until brown. Stir a couple of times while baking. Immediately loosen the nuts with a spatula before allowing them to cool. Place in an airtight container.
Makes 24 servings of 2 tablespoons each.

NOTE: These are great as snacks or sprinkled over some ice cream.

Nutrition Information per Serving	
Calories	89.03
Protein	2.10 g
Carbs	2.15 g
Fat	8.67 g
Fiber	0.88 g
Net carb	1.27 g

Mushrooms Stuffed with Asparagus Purée

½ pound fresh asparagus (about 12 spears)

1 tablespoon sour cream

½ teaspoon heavy cream

1 tablespoon olive oil

2 cloves garlic, finely minced

2 tablespoons chopped fresh parsley

1 tablespoon grated cheese (cheddar or Parmesan)

36 medium-sized fresh mushrooms

• Clean mushrooms with a small brush or paper towel and remove stems. Set aside.

• Preheat oven to 375°.

• Cut off the tips of the asparagus and chop roughly; then set aside. Cut the spears into 2″ pieces and cook in boiling water until soft, about 5 minutes. Drain well. Add cooked spears, sour cream, and heavy cream to food processor and process until smooth. Add salt & freshly ground pepper, to taste.

• In a small frying pan, heat olive oil and add garlic and asparagus tops. Sauté for 2–3 minutes and then add the parsley. Continue cooking for 1 minute.

• Grease the bottom of a glass oven-proof dish with butter. Place the mushroom caps evenly in the dish.

• Fill each mushroom cap with the asparagus purée. Add a small amount of the garlic and spear mixture to the top and sprinkle with cheese.

• Bake for 15 minutes, until the mushrooms are soft. The mushrooms may sweat a little in the oven; if they do, place them on a paper towel for just a few seconds to absorb the excess moisture, and then place on a serving dish. Serve warm.

Makes 36 pieces.

Nutrition Information per Serving	
Calories	12.74
Protein	0.89 g
Carbs	0.95 g
Fat	0.67 g
Fiber	0.35 g
Net carb	0.60 g

Party Nuts

2 egg whites
1 cup unsalted almonds
1 cup unsalted walnuts
1 cup unsalted pecans
1 cup unsalted peanuts
8 packets Splenda
1 teaspoon cinnamon
1 teaspoon cayenne pepper
½ teaspoon salt
¼ teaspoon nutmeg

- Preheat oven to 325°.
- Whisk the egg whites with the salt until foamy.
- Put the Splenda and the spices in a small bowl and blend together.
- Put the nuts in a large bowl, pour the foamy egg whites over them, and stir to coat. Sprinkle the spices over the nuts and stir well.
- Spray a cookie sheet with a nonstick agent. Spread the nuts evenly on the cookie sheet and place in the oven for approximately 15–20 minutes, until browned. The nuts need to be stirred frequently to keep from burning.
- Cool and store in an airtight container.

Makes 4 cups.

NOTE: Nutrition information is calculated on a serving size of 1/5 cup.

Nutrition Information per Serving	
Calories	159.38
Protein	4.33 g
Carbs	5.67 g
Fat	14.41 g
Fiber	1.90 g
Net carb	3.77 g

Pork Skewers

....

1 pound pork tenderloin

1 can (8 ounces) of pineapple chunks in unsweetened juice

1½ teaspoons curry powder

¼ teaspoon ground cumin

¼ teaspoon paprika

¼ teaspoon cayenne

¼ teaspoon allspice

2 tablespoons olive oil

3 tablespoons lemon juice

1 clove garlic, minced

2 tablespoons fresh minced parsley, to garnish

- Cut the tenderloin into 1½″ cubes and set aside.
- Drain the pineapple chunks and cut into 1″ cubes and set aside.
- Combine the spices in a small bowl and mix well. Add the olive oil, garlic, and lemon juice to the spice mixture to make a marinade.
- Put the tenderloin cubes in a mixing bowl, add marinade, and stir to coat. Let the pork marinate for 15–30 minutes, stirring occasionally.
- Spray a nonstick frying pan with a nonstick agent. Turn heat to medium and add pork. Cook, stirring constantly, for 8–10 minutes, until pork is done through.
- Remove from heat and thread one piece of pork with one pineapple piece on small party skewers or toothpicks. Garnish with fresh parsley.

Makes 36 pieces.

Nutrition Information per Serving	
Calories	27.03
Protein	2.56 g
Carbs	0.62 g
Fat	1.55 g
Fiber	0.08 g
Net carb	0.54 g

Salmon Ball

1 can (7.5 ounces) salmon
1 package (250 grams) cream cheese
1 tablespoon fresh lemon juice
1 green onion, finely chopped
1½ tablespoons horseradish
¼ teaspoon paprika

Topping
⅔ cup chopped walnuts
¼ cup chopped fresh parsley
2 tablespoons chopped fresh dill

- Cream together first six ingredients with a whisk, until smooth.
- Place the salmon mixture in a small cereal bowl. Cover with plastic wrap and press the wrap down to the surface of the salmon. Make a tight package. Place in the fridge overnight or for at least 2–3 hours.
- Mix together the ingredients for the topping in a large bowl.
- Remove the salmon ball from the bowl and roll it in the topping, pressing firmly.
- Place the ball on a serving plate and garnish with fresh dill stems. Serve with sliced cucumber or small low-carb crackers.
Makes approximately 2 cups.

NOTE: Nutrition information is based on 100 servings of approximately 1 teaspoon each and does not include the crackers or cucumber slices.

Thanks to my sisters, Stephanie Tompkins and Kathy Spampinato, each of whom provided ideas for this recipe.

Nutrition Information per Serving

Calories	15.96
Protein	1.14 g
Carbs	0.18 g
Fat	1.22 g
Fiber	0.03 g
Net carb	0.15 g

Spicy Chicken Wings

2 pounds chicken wings or drumettes
2 tablespoons olive oil
2 teaspoons Lawry's seasoned salt
2 teaspoons citrus & pepper seasoning
1 teaspoon paprika
1 teaspoon cayenne
1 teaspoon ground thyme

• Wash and pat dry chicken wings or drumettes and place in a bowl.
• Pour olive oil over chicken and toss to coat thoroughly.
• Blend all spices together in a small dish and then sprinkle over chicken parts and toss to coat. Use hands to rub spices into chicken skin.
• Place on a medium grill and grill 6–7 minutes a side, until done to preference. These drumettes may also be done in a 375° oven for 20 minutes, turning after about 10 minutes.
Makes 10 servings.

TIP: This recipe of spicy chicken wings is a great, if somewhat messy, appetizer. You may want to serve it with mustard dipping sauce.

Nutrition Information per Serving	
Calories	186.90
Protein	24.66 g
Carbs	0.68 g
Fat	8.87 g
Fiber	0.17 g
Net carb	0.51 g

Spicy Southern Pecans

3 cups raw pecan halves

1 large egg white

½ cup Splenda

1 tablespoon paprika

1 teaspoon cayenne pepper

½ teaspoon cinnamon

½ teaspoon nutmeg

2 teaspoons Worcestershire Sauce

- Preheat oven to 250°.
- Whisk the egg white until frothy.
- Mix the spices with the Splenda in a small bowl and blend well.
- Add the Worcestershire Sauce to the egg white and then the spices, mixing until well blended.
- Add the nuts to the egg white mixture and mix well to coat.
- Spread nuts in a single layer on a baking sheet lined with parchment paper. Pour any remaining egg mixture over nuts.
- Bake for 1–1¼ hours, until the nuts are completely dry. Stir the nuts every 20 minutes to bake evenly.

Makes 24 servings of 2 tablespoons each.

NOTE: We love these nuts, but save them for Christmas and other special occasions because it is hard not to eat them all at once.

Nutrition Information per Serving

Calories	97.97
Protein	1.53 g
Carbs	2.74 g
Fat	9.87 g
Fiber	1.41 g
Net carb	1.33 g

Sweet & Spicy Chicken Skewers

1 tablespoon soy sauce
1 tablespoon lemon juice
½ teaspoon allspice
½ teaspoon cinnamon
¼ teaspoon cayenne pepper
⅛ teaspoon paprika
½ teaspoon freshly ground pepper
2 boneless & skinless chicken breasts
½ mango
½ small pineapple

• In a shallow bowl, combine the soy sauce, lemon juice, and spices. Stir to blend well.
• Cut the chicken into 1″ square pieces and place in the bowl with sauce. Toss well to coat and let the chicken sit for 10 minutes.
• In a nonstick frying pan, over medium heat, cook the chicken until no longer pink in the middle, approximately 4–5 minutes. At this point, the chicken may be refrigerated for up to 4 hours in an airtight container.
• Cut the mango and pineapple into 1″ pieces and set aside.
• Reheat the chicken by adding a little lemon juice to the bottom of the container and heating gently in the microwave (50% power) for two 45-second bursts and stirring well after each cycle.
• Thread one piece of fruit and one piece of chicken onto individual party toothpicks.
Makes approximately 48 pieces.

Nutrition Information per Serving

Calories	10.16
Protein	1.29 g
Carbs	1.06 g
Fat	0.09 g
Fiber	0.12 g
Net carb	0.94 g

Tangy Shrimp

1 can (4.5 ounces) small shrimp

½ cup mayonnaise

2 teaspoons lemon juice

1 teaspoon tomato paste

½ teaspoon Worcestershire Sauce

2 tablespoons fresh minced parsley, divided

1 tablespoon chopped fresh chives

¼ teaspoon paprika

1 English cucumber, sliced

• Whisk together all ingredients for dressing in a small bowl, reserving 1 table-spoon of minced parsley for garnish.

• Drain shrimp and put into a small bowl. Add dressing and mix well.

• Place small amount of shrimp on cucumber slice and garnish with parsley. You may also use small crackers, although they will add considerably to the carbohydrates.

Makes 24 pieces.

Nutrition Information per Serving	
Calories	39.07
Protein	1.06 g
Carbs	0.30 g
Fat	3.70 g
Fiber	0.07 g
Net carb	0.23 g

Tuna Cheese Dip

8 ounces cream cheese, softened

6-ounce can of white tuna

2 tablespoons Sambal Oelek (chili sauce)

2 tablespoons dried parsley

2 tablespoons finely minced onion

salt & white pepper, to taste

¼ cup chopped walnuts to garnish

- Mix all ingredients (except the walnuts) with a fork until well blended. Mold into a ball in the bottom of a bowl, cover with plastic wrap, and chill in the fridge for at least 2 hours.
- Remove from bowl and roll the ball in the chopped nuts.
- Serve with fresh vegetables such as sliced zucchini and cucumber or celery and carrot sticks.

Makes 48 servings of approximately 1 teaspoon each.

NOTE: This delicious dip may also be made with shrimp or crab meat. Sambal Oelek is a ground red chili paste that you can find in the Chinese-cooking section of a grocery store.

Thanks to Nancy Cieminski of Winona, Minnesota, for this great recipe.

Nutrition Information per Serving

Calories	20.70
Protein	1.21 g
Carbs	0.16 g
Fat	1.73 g
Fiber	0.01 g
Net carb	0.15 g

SOUPS

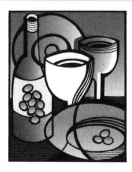

Cauliflower & Cheddar Soup

1 medium cauliflower (about 1½ pounds)
1 garlic clove, minced
1 tablespoon chopped fresh thyme
4 cups chicken broth
1 cup light cream (half & half)
1 teaspoon cornstarch
1½ cups grated sharp white cheddar cheese
½ cup finely chopped green onion
¼ teaspoon salt
freshly ground pepper, to taste

• Cut the cauliflower into small florets. Place them in a soup pot with the garlic, thyme, and chicken broth. Bring to a boil and reduce the heat to simmer and cook until the cauliflower is soft, about 10 minutes.
• Whisk the cornstarch into the light cream until dissolved. Slowly pour into the pot, stirring constantly.
• Remove the pot from the heat and remove ¾ of the soup and blend in a food processor or blender. Return the puréed soup to the soup pot with the reserved florets. Simmer, stirring occasionally, for 5–10 minutes, until the soup is slightly thickened.
• Gradually add the grated cheese, stirring constantly, until it is melted. Add the salt, pepper to taste, and green onion, reserving a few slices for garnish.
Makes 6 servings.

Nutrition Information per Serving	
Calories	226.36
Protein	12.40 g
Carbs	7.15 g
Fat	17.08 g
Fiber	1.81 g
Net carb	5.34 g

Cauliflower, Chive, & Garlic Soup

1 medium cauliflower (about 1½ pounds)

1 medium onion, minced

6 cloves garlic, minced

2 tablespoons olive oil

5 cups chicken or vegetable bouillon

½ cup heavy cream

¼ cup chopped fresh chives

2 tablespoons chopped fresh parsley

1 tablespoon chopped fresh rosemary

1 teaspoon freshly ground pepper

½ teaspoon salt

- Wash cauliflower and cut into florets.
- Warm olive oil in a large saucepan and sauté onion, garlic, parsley, salt & pepper, and rosemary until onion is soft, about 3–4 minutes. Add bouillon and cauliflower and simmer until cauliflower is soft, about 15 minutes.
- Working with batches, place vegetables and bouillon in food processor and purée.
- Return to the stove and bring to a boil. Reduce heat and gradually add heavy cream. Add all but a few of the chopped chives and heat thoroughly. Taste and adjust for salt & pepper.
- Serve with a garnish of fresh chives.
Makes 6 servings.

Nutrition Information per Serving	
Calories	137.19
Protein	1.82 g
Carbs	5.01 g
Fat	12.34 g
Fiber	0.62 g
Net carb	4.39 g

Cheesy Cabbage Soup

1 small onion, minced
1 tablespoon olive oil
1 garlic clove, minced
5 cups chicken broth
2½ cups coarsely chopped cabbage
½ cup shredded Swiss cheese
½ cup shredded white cheddar cheese
1 cup cooked ham, cubed
1 teaspoon cornstarch
1 cup heavy cream
1 cup grated carrot
1 tablespoon chopped fresh parsley
¼ teaspoon salt
freshly ground pepper, to taste

• In a large saucepan or soup pot, sauté the onion and garlic in the olive oil until just soft. Do not brown. Pour in the chicken broth, add the cabbage, parsley, and carrot, and bring to a boil. Reduce heat and simmer for 10 minutes.
• Dissolve the cornstarch in the heavy cream and add to the soup pot, stirring constantly. Gradually stir in the cheese until melted. Add the cubed ham and salt & pepper, to taste. Simmer for an additional 5 minutes, stirring occasionally.
Makes 6 servings.

Nutrition Information per Serving	
Calories	318.24
Protein	13.64 g
Carbs	7.39 g
Fat	26.54 g
Fiber	1.46 g
Net carb	5.93 g

Chicken Soup

4 boneless chicken breasts
6 cups chicken bouillon
2 cups water
4 celery stalks with leaves
1 teaspoon salt
2 teaspoons freshly ground
  pepper
2 teaspoons butter
½ cup minced onion

1 cup finely chopped celery
2 cups shredded green cabbage
½ cup sliced fresh mushrooms
2 cups chopped fresh vegetables
  (broccoli or cauliflower florets
  or green beans, asparagus,
  etc.)
1 medium carrot, thinly sliced

• Place 2 cups of bouillon, chicken breasts, and celery stalks in a large saucepan over medium-high heat. Bring to a boil and reduce heat. Cover and simmer for 20–25 minutes, until chicken is cooked through. Remove breasts and set aside. Remove celery stalks and discard.
• Strain liquid 2 or 3 times until clear. You can strain this liquid through a paper coffee filter to catch the fat. Reserve liquid and set aside.
• Melt butter in a large saucepan over medium heat. Add onions and mushrooms and sauté for 3–4 minutes.
• Add reserved liquid plus 4 cups of additional chicken bouillon. Add all vegetables, cover, and simmer for at least 1 hour. Add water if the soup appears to be getting too thick.
• Cut the chicken into bite-sized pieces and add them to the pot 20 minutes before serving.
Makes 6 servings.

Nutrition Information per Serving	
Calories	155.33
Protein	22.30 g
Carbs	7.04 g
Fat	3.63 g
Fiber	1.47 g
Net carb	5.57 g

Chunky Ham Soup

1 cup diced cooked ham
2 tablespoons light olive oil
2 garlic cloves, minced
1½ tablespoons chopped fresh parsley
1 medium sweet onion, minced
8 cups chicken or beef stock
4 large celery sticks, cut into ½″ pieces
1 cup sliced mushrooms
2 cups sliced cabbage
1 cup trimmed green beans
1 cup asparagus spears, cut into 1″ pieces
1 medium carrot, thinly sliced

• Heat olive oil over medium heat in a large soup pot. Add the onion and garlic and sauté for about 3–4 minutes. Add the mushrooms and parsley and continue cooking for 3 or 4 more minutes, until the mushrooms are soft.
• Add the chicken (or beef) stock and the cabbage, beans, carrots, and cauliflower. Simmer for approximately 1 hour.
• Add the diced ham, asparagus, and celery and continue to simmer for 15 minutes.
Makes 4 servings.

TIP: This soup may be refrigerated and reheated before serving.

Nutrition Information per Serving

Calories	202.90
Protein	12.13 g
Carbs	10.99 g
Fat	13.34 g
Fiber	4.02 g
Net carb	6.97 g

Cream of Cauliflower Soup

1½ pounds fresh cauliflower
2 tablespoons butter
4 cups chicken bouillon
1 medium sweet onion, minced
1 cup light cream (half & half)
½ cup heavy cream
1 tablespoon chopped fresh
  thyme
1 tablespoon chopped fresh
  parsley

1 teaspoon freshly ground
  pepper
½ teaspoon salt
½ teaspoon paprika

To Finish
¼ cup shredded cheddar cheese
1 tablespoon chopped fresh
  parsley

• In a large saucepan, over medium heat, sauté onion in butter for 2–3 minutes. Add herbs and continue cooking for 1 minute, stirring constantly. Add chicken broth and cauliflower that has been cut into small pieces. Cover and simmer until cauliflower is soft, about 15 minutes.
• Process in batches in a food processor until smooth. Return to soup pot and gradually add the creams, paprika, and salt & pepper. Heat thoroughly, but do not boil.
• Garnish with shredded cheese and a sprinkle of chopped fresh parsley.
Makes 6 servings.

TIP: This soup may be made 2–3 hours before serving. Refrigerate and reheat before serving. Also good when reheated the next day.

Nutrition Information per Serving

Calories	229.69
Protein	5.25 g
Carbs	5.29 g
Fat	21.11 g
Fiber	0.56 g
Net carb	4.73 g

Cream of Mushroom Soup

2 cups fresh mushrooms, cleaned and finely chopped
3 tablespoons olive oil
1 small red onion, finely chopped
4 cups chicken bouillon
1 tablespoon flour
salt & freshly ground pepper, to taste
1 bay leaf
1 teaspoon Fine Herbs

To Finish
1 cup heavy cream
chopped fresh parsley

• Heat olive oil in heavy saucepan. Cook onions and mushrooms for about 5 minutes, stirring constantly. Add flour and continue cooking for 1 minute.
• Gradually add chicken bouillon, herbs, and bay leaf while stirring constantly. Bring to a boil, lower heat, and cover. Gently simmer for 20 minutes.
• Remove the saucepan from the heat. Remove the bay leaf. Adjust salt & pepper to taste.
• To finish, gradually add the heavy cream and return to medium heat to heat through. Garnish each serving with chopped fresh parsley.
Makes 4 servings.

Nutrition Information per Serving

Calories	339.26
Protein	3.63 g
Carbs	8.92 g
Fat	33.49 g
Fiber	1.22 g
Net carb	7.70 g

Creamy Asparagus Soup

2 pounds fresh asparagus
2 cups vegetable bouillon
2 teaspoons olive oil
2 small onions, minced
2 cloves garlic, minced
1 cup light cream (half & half)
½ cup heavy cream

1 tablespoon lemon zest

To Finish
2 tablespoons sour cream
1 teaspoon heavy cream
freshly ground pepper, to taste

• Wash and pat dry asparagus spears. Cut off tough ends, cut 1″ tip off each, and reserve. Cut remaining spears into 2″ pieces.
• Bring vegetable bouillon to a boil. Add asparagus spears and cook for approximately 5 minutes. Strain asparagus into a bowl, reserving ¾ cup of broth.
• Heat oil in a pan over medium heat. Add onion and garlic and sauté for 5 minutes. Add asparagus stalks and cream and simmer 8 minutes, until tender.
• Combine asparagus mixture with reserved broth and process in a blender until smooth. This is a thick and creamy soup.
• Steam asparagus tips for 2–3 minutes, until tender.
• Combine asparagus purée and lemon zest. Simmer over low heat until warmed through.
• To finish, serve into individual bowls and add asparagus tips and a swirl of sour cream blended with the heavy cream and freshly ground pepper. *Makes 4 servings.*

TIP: The sour cream will lighten up, so that it floats, if blended with a bit of heavy cream or water before being used.

Nutrition Information per Serving

Calories	326.88
Protein	6.94 g
Carbs	11.69 g
Fat	28.59 g
Fiber	3.82 g
Net carb	7.87 g

Creamy Broccoli Soup

1½ pounds fresh broccoli
    florets
4 tablespoons butter
4 cups chicken bouillon
1 medium sweet onion, minced
1 cup light cream (half & half)
½ cup heavy cream
1 tablespoon chopped fresh
    thyme
1 tablespoon chopped fresh
    chives

1 teaspoon freshly ground
    pepper
½ teaspoon salt
½ teaspoon ground cumin

To Finish
2 tablespoons sour cream
1 teaspoon heavy cream
1 teaspoon chopped fresh
    parsley

• In a large saucepan, over medium heat, sauté onion in butter for 2–3 minutes, until soft. Add herbs and continue cooking 1 minute longer, stirring constantly. Add chicken bouillon and broccoli florets, cut into small pieces. Cover and simmer until broccoli is soft, about 15 minutes.
• Process in batches in a food processor until smooth.
• Return to soup pot and gradually add the creams, cumin, and salt & pepper. Heat thoroughly but do not boil.
• To finish, garnish individual servings with sour cream that has been blended with heavy cream so that it swirls on the soup and a sprinkle of chopped fresh parsley.
Makes 8 servings.

TIP: This soup may be made 2–3 hours before serving. Refrigerate and reheat before serving. Also good when reheated the next day.

Nutrition Information per Serving

Calories	186.73
Protein	2.07 g
Carbs	4.23 g
Fat	18.52 g
Fiber	0.33 g
Net carb	3.90 g

French Onion Soup

1 pound onions (4 cups sliced)
¼ cup butter
3 cloves garlic, minced
6 cups beef bouillon
½ teaspoon salt
freshly ground pepper, to taste
1½ cups shredded mozzarella

• Mince the garlic and cut whole, peeled onions into thin rounds.
• Melt butter in a large soup pot and add the onion and garlic. Caramelize the onion by cooking it over medium heat until the natural sugar is released and the onion turns brown and is reduced in volume. This will take about 25–30 minutes, during which time the mixture should be stirred frequently.
• Add the beef bouillon and salt & freshly ground black pepper; then reduce heat and simmer for 35 minutes.
• To serve, pour the soup into 4 oven-proof soup bowls. Sprinkle each bowl with shredded cheese, and place all 4 bowls on a cookie sheet.
• Place the cookie sheet under a hot broiler for 2–3 minutes, until the cheese is melted and has browned.
Makes 4 servings.

NOTE: If you are worried about the fat content of this soup, reduce the amount of shredded cheese that you use for finishing the soup.

Thanks to my sister Kathy Spampinato, who provided the basic recipe for this soup.

Nutrition Information per Serving

Calories	359.76
Protein	20.58 g
Carbs	10.58 g
Fat	26.66 g
Fiber	1.41 g
Net carb	9.17 g

Gazpacho Soup

4 cups tomato juice

4 medium tomatoes

2 tablespoons olive oil

2 tablespoons red wine vinegar

1 small red onion, quartered

½ medium sweet green pepper

½ medium cucumber

1 stalk celery, chopped

1 clove garlic, chopped

1 tablespoon each chopped
fresh parsley and thyme

1 teaspoon freshly ground
pepper

½ teaspoon salt

1 tablespoon sour cream

½ teaspoon heavy cream

chopped fresh parsley, to
garnish

• Peel skins from the tomatoes and cut into wedges. Cut cucumber in half lengthwise, remove seeds, and cut into 1″ pieces.
• Working with batches, put half the vegetables and half the tomato juice and other ingredients into a food processor and blend until smooth.
• Put batches together in a large bowl and chill. Remove from fridge 5 minutes before serving. If the soup is very thick, you may add some more tomato juice.
• Blend the sour cream with a small amount of heavy cream to lighten consistency.
• To serve, spoon soup into individual bowls, swirl sour cream mixture on top, and add a sprinkle of chopped parsley.
Makes 6 servings.

NOTE: This is a wonderful soup on a hot night, and it looks gorgeous with the sour cream and parsley.

Thanks to my good friend Kathleen Costello, who provided the basic recipe, which I adjusted.

Nutrition Information per Serving	
Calories	94.98
Protein	2.20 g
Carbs	12.07 g
Fat	5.49 g
Fiber	1.75 g
Net carb	10.32 g

Hearty Vegetable Soup

2 tablespoons light olive oil
2 cloves garlic, minced
1½ tablespoons chopped fresh parsley
1 medium sweet onion, minced
8 cups chicken or beef stock
4 large celery sticks, cut into ½″ pieces
1 cup sliced mushrooms
2 cups sliced cabbage
1 cup trimmed green beans
1 cup asparagus spears, cut into 1″ pieces
1 cup cauliflower florets
1 medium zucchini, cut into ½″ pieces
1 medium carrot, thinly sliced

• Heat olive oil over medium heat in a large soup pot. Add the onion and garlic and sauté for about 3–4 minutes. Add the mushrooms and parsley and continue cooking for 3 or 4 more minutes, until the mushrooms are soft.
• Add the chicken (or beef) stock and the cabbage, beans, carrots, and cauliflower. Simmer for approximately 1 hour.
• Add the asparagus, celery, and zucchini and continue to simmer for 15 minutes.
Makes 4 servings.

TIP: This soup may be refrigerated and reheated before serving.

Nutrition Information per Serving	
Calories	117.89
Protein	3.78 g
Carbs	12.16 g
Fat	7.52 g
Fiber	4.85 g
Net carb	7.31 g

Meatball Soup

1–1½ pounds extra lean ground beef

1 egg

2 tablespoons bread crumbs

½ teaspoon ground black pepper

¼ teaspoon salt

2 tablespoons olive oil

½ cup diced onion

1 cup sliced mushrooms

4 cups chopped cabbage

2 cloves garlic, minced

3 medium carrots, chopped

6 cups beef broth

• Combine the ground beef with beaten egg, bread crumbs, and salt & pepper.

• Heat olive oil over medium heat in a large soup pot. Form beef mixture into ½″ balls and brown on all sides. You may have to do this in lots, depending on the size of your pot. Remove meatballs and set aside.

• Add onion and mushrooms and sauté for 5 minutes or until soft. Be sure to scrape the bottom of the pan to loosen any brown bits since they add to the flavor. Add ½ cup of the beef broth and continue to work away at the brown bits on the bottom.

• Add the remaining 5½ cups of beef broth into the pot. Carefully add the meatballs back into the pot. Stir in the chopped carrots and cabbage. You may want to add a little extra freshly ground pepper & salt at this point. Reduce heat and simmer, covered, for 1 or 2 hours.

Makes 6–8 servings.

NOTE: Nutrition information is calculated based on 1 1/2 pounds of ground beef and 6 servings of soup.

Thanks to Mary Sinclair of Thunder Bay, Ontario, who provided the inspiration for this soup.

Nutrition Information per Serving

Calories	329.21
Protein	26.18 g
Carbs	9.69 g
Fat	20.77 g
Fiber	2.67 g
Net carb	7.02 g

Summer Squash Soup

3 yellow summer squash (yellow zucchini)
1 tablespoon olive oil
1 large sweet onion, minced
3 cloves garlic, minced
3 sprigs lemon thyme (or 6 sprigs thyme and 3 strips lemon peel)
2 cups chicken bouillon

zest & juice of a lemon
¼ teaspoon salt
freshly ground pepper, to taste

To Finish
2 tablespoons sour cream
1 teaspoon heavy cream
2 teaspoons lemon zest
4 small sprigs lemon thyme

• Wash and trim ends of squash. Cut off any blemishes on the skins. Chop coarsely into approximately 1″ pieces and set aside.
• In a large saucepan, heat olive oil over medium heat. Add onions and garlic and sauté for 3–4 minutes or until onions are soft.
• Add squash and lemon thyme and cook, stirring constantly, for about 5 minutes.
• Increase heat to medium-high. Add chicken bouillon and salt. Cook at a low boil for 20 minutes or until squash is soft.
• Remove from heat and discard the lemon thyme. Purée in batches in a blender and return to saucepan to heat thoroughly. Add the juice of a lemon.
• To finish, serve with a garnish of sour cream, a sprinkle of lemon zest, and a sprig of thyme or lemon thyme.
Makes 4 servings.

TIP: The sour cream will lighten up so that it floats if you mix it with a bit of heavy cream or water before you use it as a garnish.

Nutrition Information per Serving	
Calories	87.77
Protein	2.75 g
Carbs	12.27 g
Fat	4.24 g
Fiber	3.68 g
Net carb	8.59 g

Tomato, Herb, & Curried Chicken Soup

2 boneless, skinless chicken breasts

3 tablespoons extra virgin olive oil

¼ teaspoon mustard seeds

¼ teaspoon ground cumin

2 teaspoons curry powder

¼ cup heavy cream

4 cloves garlic, minced

½ sweet onion, minced

1 cup chicken bouillon

4 large, ripe tomatoes, roughly chopped

4 packets Splenda

2 tablespoons chopped fresh flat leaf parsley

2 tablespoons chopped fresh rosemary

1 tablespoon chopped fresh chives

fresh chives for garnish

freshly ground pepper

• Heat 2 tablespoons of olive oil in a soup pot or large stew pot. Add the minced onion and garlic and sauté for 2–3 minutes. Add the fresh herbs and continue cooking for 1 minute.

• Add the tomatoes (these should be roughly chopped into 1″ pieces) and Splenda and simmer, stirring frequently, for approximately 15–20 minutes, until cooked through and soft.

• Prepare the chicken while the tomatoes are simmering. Cut the chicken into ½″ pieces.

continued

- Heat 1 tablespoon of the olive oil in a nonstick frying pan. Add the chicken and sauté over medium heat until browned on all sides. Remove chicken from the pan and set aside.
- Add the mustard seed, cumin, and curry to the pan. Add the heavy cream and stir to blend. Add back the chicken with any juices and stir for a minute to coat. Turn off heat and set aside.
- Take approximately ¾ of the tomato mixture, put it into a food processor, and blend until smooth.
- Return the tomato mixture to the soup pot and add the chicken bouillon, stirring to blend. You now have a mostly creamy tomato base, with a few chunky pieces to add texture.
- Add the chicken with the curry sauce to the soup, stirring to blend the sauce with the soup. Season with freshly ground pepper and simmer for 15 minutes to allow the flavors to blend.
- Serve with a couple of fresh chives floating on the soup and a sprinkle of freshly ground pepper.

Makes 4 servings.

NOTE: The inspiration for this really delicious soup came from a lovely country inn just outside Queenstown, New Zealand. I thought about this soup for months, making constant notes, before trying to put it together. It took more than a couple of trials, but the result is well worth it, I think.

Nutrition Information per Serving

Calories	163.75
Protein	13.82 g
Carbs	5.42 g
Fat	8.97 g
Fiber	1.44 g
Net carb	3.98 g

Turkey Broth

1 turkey carcass
4–5 quarts water
1 onion, quartered
1 carrot, cut up
6 celery tops with leaves
salt & pepper, to taste

• Place the carcass in a large soup or stew pot with sufficient water to cover the carcass.
• Add the carrot, onion, and celery tops. Cover pot and simmer for 2–3 hours.
• Strain the broth 2 or 3 times to eliminate the bones, vegetables, and other bits.
• Cool in the fridge overnight. Remove from fridge and skim off any fat that may have solidified on top.

Makes 4–5 quarts of turkey broth, depending on size of carcass and amount of water used.

NOTE: Nutrition calculation is for the entire batch of broth. Make your own chicken broth using essentially the same recipe and substituting one or more chicken carcasses.

Nutrition Information per Serving	
Calories	117.77
Protein	14.34 g
Carbs	2.39 g
Fat	5.33 g
Fiber	0.57 g
Net carb	1.82 g

Turkey Soup

3–4 quarts turkey broth (see previous page)
1 medium sweet onion, minced
6–8 medium carrots, thinly sliced
2 cups cauliflower florets
2 cups green beans, cut into ½″ pieces
4 cups green cabbage, cut into 1″ pieces
2 cups chopped celery
4 cups bite-sized cooked turkey meat
salt & freshly ground pepper, to taste

• Pour turkey broth into a large soup pot with a lid. Add prepared vegetables and salt & pepper.
• Simmer, covered, for at least 2 hours. The cauliflower will break up and become almost like barley. The cabbage replaces rice and provides extra bulk and flavor.
• One hour before serving, add the turkey meat, cover, and continue to simmer. Taste for seasoning at this point and add more salt & pepper if needed.
Makes 8–10 servings.

NOTE: This is a delicious, filling soup. It is a meal on its own. The soup freezes well or will stay fresh in the fridge for a couple of days.

Nutrition Information per Serving	
Calories	200.69
Protein	19.90 g
Carbs	12.96 g
Fat	7.77 g
Fiber	4.03 g
Net carb	8.93 g

SALADS

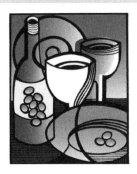

NOTE: The nutrition information for salads includes the nutrition value of the recommended dressing unless otherwise noted in the recipe.

Broccoli Salad

3 cups broccoli florets
2 green onions, chopped
1 cup sliced fresh mushrooms
¼ cup roasted pine nuts
½ green pepper, cut into matchsticks

Dressing
½ cup mayonnaise
1 packet Splenda
3 tablespoons rice wine vinegar

• Steam florets for 2–3 minutes, until tender crisp and bright green. Plunge into ice water to stop cooking process. Strain and pat dry. Add other ingredients in a large mixing bowl.
• Whisk together dressing ingredients. Pour over salad and mix well. Chill for at least an hour before serving.
Makes 4 servings.

TIP: You may substitute either sweet red pepper or yellow pepper for the green pepper, and this adds a nice note of color.

Nutrition Information per Serving

Calories	235.12
Protein	2.41 g
Carbs	6.41 g
Fat	22.30 g
Fiber	0.76 g
Net carb	5.65 g

Chicken Salad

4 boneless, skinless chicken breasts
2 cups chicken bouillon
4 celery stalks with leaves
1 cup finely diced celery
½ cup roasted whole, blanched almonds
½ medium sweet red pepper, cut into matchsticks

Dressing
½ cup real mayonnaise
4 teaspoons lemon juice
4–6 teaspoons reserved poaching liquid

• Poach the chicken breasts with the celery stalks in the bouillon for 15–20 minutes, until completely cooked. Remove from stove top and reserve liquid. The reserved liquid needs to be strained. A paper coffee filter fitted in the strainer works well for straining the fat from the liquid. Put the reserved liquid aside. Place the chicken breasts in the fridge to cool.
• Toast the almonds (this can be done in a nonstick frying pan, stirring constantly, or in the oven at 350° for 10–15 minutes, turning every 5 minutes) and let cool. Chop the celery and red pepper and set aside.
• To make the dressing, add the lemon juice and reserved liquid to the mayonnaise until desired consistency is obtained. You may need a little more reserved liquid, depending on desired thickness of dressing.

continued

• Remove the chicken from the fridge and cut into bite-sized pieces. Put chicken, almonds, celery, and red pepper in a large bowl and mix with dressing until well coated. This salad will keep in a covered bowl in the fridge for up to 2 days.

Makes 6 servings.

NOTE: This recipe comes from my good friend Pearl Rudin in Toronto, Ontario. Pearl says that originally it came from an old *New York Times* cookbook and that she adjusted it slightly. I made some further minor revisions to Pearl's version.

TIP: A nice variation is to replace the reserved liquid with raspberry vinegar in the dressing. This provides some tang and a bit of color to the dressing.

Nutrition Information per Serving

Calories	309.89
Protein	22.67 g
Carbs	4.21 g
Fat	22.20 g
Fiber	1.80 g
Net carb	2.41 g

Chicken with Pineapple

2 cups cooked white chicken meat, cut up
2 green onions, chopped
2 celery stalks, finely minced
½ cup unsalted cashews, coarsely chopped
¼ cup pineapple chunks, chopped
Curried Pineapple Dressing (see recipe)

• Cut the chicken into bite-sized pieces and mix together with other ingredients in a bowl. (I use canned pineapple chunks in unsweetened pineapple juice. I drain the chunks, reserving the liquid for use in the dressing, and cut the chunks into smaller pieces.)
• Combine the chicken with the dressing and mix well.
• Serve on a bed of red leaf lettuce, with a couple of cherry tomatoes for color.
Makes 4 servings.

TIP: Two large boneless, skinless breasts that have been poached work well for this salad.

Nutrition Information per Serving

Calories	385.16
Protein	17.38 g
Carbs	9.63 g
Fat	30.77 g
Fiber	1.01 g
Net carb	8.62 g

Crab Salad

....

8 ounces crab meat
2 medium tomatoes
1 medium red onion, thinly sliced in rounds
16 fresh asparagus spears
6 cups green leaf lettuce
Dijon Vinaigrette (see recipe)

• Wash asparagus and cut tough ends off. Place in boiling water for 2–3 minutes, until tender crisp. Drain and plunge into ice water until cool. Wrap in paper towel and set aside.
• Divide the lettuce evenly and arrange in an attractive layer on each plate. Layer the ingredients as follows: tomato, separated onion rings, and 4 asparagus spears across the top of each salad.
• Drizzle the salad with the Dijon Vinaigrette. Sprinkle the crab meat across the top of the asparagus.

Makes 4 servings.

Nutrition Information per Serving	
Calories	267.82
Protein	15.16 g
Carbs	9.55 g
Fat	20.08 g
Fiber	2.58 g
Net carb	6.97 g

Cucumber Salad

1 small English cucumber
1 small green or sweet red pepper

Dressing
¼ cup white wine vinegar
1 tablespoon olive oil
1 teaspoon dry mustard
1 teaspoon chopped fresh parsley

• Thinly slice the cucumber. Cut green pepper into matchstick pieces.
• Whisk together dressing ingredients and toss with vegetables. Serve chilled.
Makes 4 servings.

Nutrition Information per Serving

Calories	55.16
Protein	0.81 g
Carbs	4.90 g
Fat	3.66 g
Fiber	1.17 g
Net carb	3.73 g

Curried Chicken Salad

2 cups cooked white chicken meat, cut up
2 green onions, chopped
2 celery stalks, finely minced
⅓ cup unsalted cashews, coarsely chopped
¼ cup seedless raisins
Lemon Curry Dressing (see recipe)

• Cut the chicken into bite-sized pieces and mix with other ingredients in a bowl.
• Combine the chicken with dressing and mix well.
• Serve on a bed of leaf lettuce, with some sliced cucumber for contrast.
Makes 4 servings.

NOTE: The raisins really add to the carbo-hydrate count. They can be reduced, and the carbohydrate count will fall.

TIP: Two large boneless, skinless breasts that have been poached work well for this salad.

Nutrition Information per Serving

Calories	369.80
Protein	16.88 g
Carbs	12.55 g
Fat	28.15 g
Fiber	1.34 g
Net carb	11.21 g

Curried Mango Salad

6 cups mixed greens
1 ripe mango, diced
½ cup whole roasted cashews
2 chopped green onions
Curried Red Wine Dressing (see recipe)

• Wash and wipe dry all greens. Add mango and onion to the greens. Keep cashews in a separate small dish until ready to dress.
• Dress the salad with the Curried Red Wine Dressing just before serving.
Makes 6 servings if used as an appetizer or 4 lunch-sized servings.

NOTE: Nutrition information is calculated based on 6 servings.

TIP: To reduce the grams of carbohydrates, use just half a mango. This fruit is delicious but high in carbs. You can also substitute papaya for the mango to reduce the carb content. I always use fresh baby spinach as part of my greens to increase the fiber in the salad.

Nutrition Information per Serving	
Calories	270.40
Protein	4.98 g
Carbs	13.74 g
Fat	23.28 g
Fiber	3.90 g
Net carb	9.84 g

Thanks to my good friend Jacqueline McDonald of Toronto, Ontario, for this recipe, which I adapted slightly.

Easy Coleslaw

4 cups finely sliced green cabbage
2 cups finely sliced red cabbage

Dressing
½ cup real mayonnaise
1½ tablespoons lemon juice
1 tablespoon lime juice

• Whisk together dressing ingredients in a small bowl. Combine dressing with cabbage in a large bowl and mix well.
• Chill for at least an hour before serving to allow flavors to blend. Will keep up to 48 hours in a fridge.
Makes 8 servings.

TIP: To keep the red color from running, rinse the sliced red cabbage under cold water in a colander, until the water runs clear.

Nutrition Information per Serving

Calories	114.36
Protein	0.76 g
Carbs	3.28 g
Fat	12.14 g
Fiber	1.17 g
Net carb	2.11 g

Egg Salad

4 hard-boiled eggs
1 celery stick, finely minced
1 green onion, finely chopped
¼ cup red or green pepper, finely minced
⅔ cup mayonnaise
1½ teaspoons Dijon mustard
½ teaspoon salt
freshly ground pepper, to taste
6–8 red lettuce leaves

• Place 4 eggs in a pot and cover with water. Bring to a boil, reduce heat, and boil for 10 minutes. Rinse the eggs in cold water to cool them and place them in the fridge for at least an hour.
• Crack the eggshells and peel off. Roughly chop the eggs. Add the celery, onion, and red or green pepper.
• Mix the mayonnaise, mustard, and salt & pepper. Add the dressing to the egg mixture and mix gently until just blended.
• Serve on a bed of red lettuce.
Makes 2–3 servings.

Nutrition Information per Serving	
Calories	293.68
Protein	9.61 g
Carbs	2.79 g
Fat	28.04 g
Fiber	0.46 g
Net carb	2.33 g

Fancy Coleslaw

6 cups finely sliced green cabbage
1 cup finely sliced red cabbage
1 medium carrot, finely shredded
½ medium sweet red pepper, cut into matchsticks

Dressing
½ cup real mayonnaise
1 tablespoon lemon juice
1 tablespoon white wine vinegar
1 packet Splenda

- Whisk together dressing ingredients.
- Wash and prepare vegetables and put in a large bowl. Add dressing to vegetables and combine well.
- Chill for at least an hour before serving to allow flavors to blend. Will keep up to 48 hours in a fridge.

Makes 8 servings.

TIP: To keep the red color from running, rinse the sliced red cabbage under cold water in a colander, until the water runs clear.

Nutrition Information per Serving	
Calories	123.07
Protein	1.09 g
Carbs	5.33 g
Fat	12.20 g
Fiber	1.85 g
Net carb	3.48 g

Grapefruit & Spinach Salad

1 pound fresh baby spinach (about 8 cups)
2 fresh pink grapefruits
½ cup toasted almond slivers
Creamy White Wine Vinaigrette (see recipe)

• Wash the spinach and remove stems. Place on paper towels to dry. Tear into bite-sized pieces and place in a large bowl.
• Peel the grapefruit and separate into natural sections. Peel the sections and cut into ½" pieces.
• Add the grapefruit to the spinach and toss. Add the almonds and dressing just before serving.

Makes 4 lunch-sized servings or 6 appetizer salads.

NOTE: Nutrition calculation is based on 6 servings. This is a delicious new twist on a spinach salad. It is great as an appetizer at dinner or as a lunch salad.

Nutrition Information per Serving

Calories	103.60
Protein	4.25 g
Carbs	9.96 g
Fat	6.34 g
Fiber	3.24 g
Net carb	6.72 g

Green Bean & Almond Salad

3 cups green beans (about 1 pound)
½ cup roasted almond pieces
1 medium sweet red pepper, cut into matchsticks
White Wine Vinaigrette (see recipe)

• Wash and trim the beans. Cut into 2–3″ pieces. Plunge beans into boiling water and leave for 3–4 minutes, until bright green and crispy tender. Drain and immediately put into a large bowl of ice water. Strain and pat dry.
• Put the beans, almond pieces, and red pepper into a large bowl.
• Pour dressing over vegetables. Stir well to blend flavors. Serve chilled.
Makes 6 servings.

Nutrition Information per Serving

Calories	188.81
Protein	3.26 g
Carbs	7.85 g
Fat	17.27 g
Fiber	3.29 g
Net carb	4.56 g

Greens with Pecans & Blue Cheese

6 cups washed, mixed baby greens
½ cup roasted pecan halves
4 ounces blue cheese
Creamy Raspberry Vinaigrette (see recipe)

• Clean and trim greens and place in a large salad bowl. Toss greens with Creamy Raspberry Vinaigrette dressing.
• Arrange greens on 4 salad plates. Sprinkle with pecan halves, evenly divided among the servings. Crumble blue cheese on top of the greens.
Makes 4 servings.

Nutrition Information per Serving

Calories	331.82
Protein	8.24 g
Carbs	5.38 g
Fat	32.11 g
Fiber	2.47 g
Net carb	2.91 g

Grilled Asparagus Salad

6 cups wild greens
16 asparagus spears
1 small sweet red pepper
½ small sweet yellow pepper
2 tablespoons olive oil
½ teaspoon freshly ground pepper
¼ cup toasted pecans, chopped
Balsamic Vinaigrette (see recipe)

• Preheat grill to medium heat. Cut peppers into quarters and remove all seeds
and extra pulp. Brush asparagus and peppers with olive oil and sprinkle
asparagus with some freshly ground pepper. Grill over medium heat for 3–4
minutes a side, watching carefully. You want the vegetables to be soft and have
grill marks without being overdone. Set aside to cool.
• Clean greens and slice grilled peppers. Mix together in a large bowl.
• Toss together the vinaigrette and greens, reserving a small amount of dressing.
• Divide salad evenly among 4 plates. Arrange the asparagus spears attractively
on top of the greens, sprinkle with toasted pecans, and drizzle with the
remaining dressing.
Makes 4 servings.

**Nutrition Information
per Serving**

Calories	180.23
Protein	4.16 g
Carbs	11.76 g
Fat	14.52 g
Fiber	4.02 g
Net carb	7.74 g

Grilled Chicken Salad

4 boneless, skinless chicken breasts
½ cup marinade (orange, lemon herb, or other)
6 cups mixed fresh greens
2 hard-boiled eggs
4 celery stalks, chopped
4 ounces cheese cut into bite-sized pieces (brie or similar type)
½ medium sweet red pepper, thinly sliced
½ cucumber, thinly sliced
¼ cup toasted almond slices
Creamy Raspberry Vinaigrette (or other dressing of choice)

• Marinate chicken breasts in a shallow bowl for at least 30 minutes.
• Preheat grill to medium high. (Breasts may also be done in a medium-hot frying pan with 1 tablespoon of olive oil.)
• Clean greens and distribute evenly among 4 plates. Cut eggs into slices and arrange around the perimeter of each plate.
• Divide and arrange the cheese and other vegetables attractively on top of the greens.
• Grill (or fry) the chicken breasts for 4–5 minutes on each side, until cooked through. Remove from heat and slice into thin slices, on the diagonal.
• Pour dressing over greens and place sliced hot chicken on top of greens. Sprinkle with toasted almond slivers.

Makes 4 servings.

Nutrition Information per Serving

Calories	454.96
Protein	44.79 g
Carbs	10.91 g
Fat	26.28 g
Fiber	3.88 g
Net carb	7.03 g

Marinated Veggies

....

2 cups broccoli florets
2 cups cauliflower florets
1 English cucumber with peel, quartered and sliced
2 cups celery, diced
1 medium sweet red pepper, chopped
1 medium sweet yellow pepper, chopped
1 cup carrot, sliced or julienned
Creamy Vegetable Marinade (see recipe)

- Wash, pat dry, and cut all vegetables.
- Put vegetables in a large bowl and pour marinade over them. Stir well to coat. Place in fridge for at least a couple of hours before serving.
Makes 8 servings.

VARIATION: This is a great salad that can have many variations by adding any vegetable you like. Keep in mind that some veggies have more carbs than others. To keep your carb content down, add asparagus, green onions, mushrooms, or green beans.

NOTE: This salad will keep for 2–3 days in an airtight container in the fridge.

Nutrition Information per Serving

Calories	167.26
Protein	2.19 g
Carbs	9.15 g
Fat	14.44 g
Fiber	2.34 g
Net carb	6.81 g

Oriental Chicken Salad

2 cooked boneless chicken breasts (use Orange Chicken)
4 cups shredded iceberg lettuce
4 cups chopped or shredded green cabbage
4 small green onions, chopped
1 cup chopped or shredded bok choy
½ small sweet red pepper, thinly sliced
1 cup bean sprouts
½ cup mandarin orange pieces
½ cup toasted almond slivers
1 teaspoon sesame seeds, to garnish
Soy Ginger Dressing (see recipe)

• Roughly chop lettuce, cabbage, and bok choy and place in a large bowl. Slice green onion and red pepper and add to bowl.
• Cut cooked chicken into bite-sized pieces and set aside.
• Add mandarin orange sections to bowl, along with roasted almond slivers and bean sprouts. Mix all ingredients.
• Toss the salad with Soy Ginger Dressing.
• Divide the salad evenly among 4 plates. Place chicken pieces on top and sprinkle with sesame seeds.
Makes 4 servings.

Nutrition Information per Serving	
Calories	333.60
Protein	37.84 g
Carbs	17.19 g
Fat	10.94 g
Fiber	5.61 g
Net carb	11.58 g

Oriental Coleslaw

1 cup green cabbage, chopped
3 cups napa cabbage, chopped
2 cups red cabbage, chopped
1 carrot, grated
½ cup thinly sliced red onion
Oriental Dressing (see recipe)

• Wash and cut all vegetables and combine in a large bowl.
• Toss the slaw with the dressing, cover, and chill in the fridge for an hour to allow the flavors to blend.
Makes 6–8 servings.

NOTE: Nutrition information is calculated based on 8 servings. This is a really fun and tasty variation on coleslaw. The hot note in the dressing is a surprise. As with the other varieties, it will keep well in the fridge for 2–3 days.

TIP: To prevent the red color from running, rinse the sliced red cabbage under cold water in a colander, until the water runs clear.

Nutrition Information per Serving	
Calories	99.51
Protein	1.40 g
Carbs	6.69 g
Fat	8.21 g
Fiber	1.89 g
Net Fiber	4.80 g

Salmon Salad

2 cups cooked, cut-up salmon
2 green onions, finely chopped
2 celery stalks, finely diced

Dressing
½ cup mayonnaise
3 teaspoons fresh lemon juice
2 packets Splenda
1 tablespoon chopped fresh dill
½ teaspoon freshly ground pepper

• Cut salmon into bite-sized pieces and put into a bowl with onion and celery.
• Whisk together all dressing ingredients in a small bowl. Pour dressing over salmon and mix well.
• Serve over a bed of butter lettuce.
Makes 4 servings.

Nutrition Information per Serving	
Calories	352.13
Protein	22.46 g
Carbs	2.61 g
Fat	29.25 g
Fiber	0.56 g
Net carb	2.05 g

Salmon & Avocado Salad

juice of half a lemon
2 ripe avocados
2 chopped green onions
½ cup diced celery
½ cup diced red pepper
1 can (7.5 ounces) of salmon (or cooked fresh salmon if available)
2 tablespoons mayonnaise
¼ teaspoon salt
chopped fresh dill

- Squeeze half a lemon and put juice in a bowl.
- Cut avocados in half lengthwise and dispose of pits. Scoop avocado out of the shells and set shells aside. Dice the avocado into very small pieces and place pieces in lemon juice. Stir well to coat to prevent browning.
- Add the green onion, celery, and red pepper.
- Mash the salmon well (including bones, if you like) and add to the avocado mixture. Add salt and chopped fresh dill, to taste.
- Add the mayonnaise and stir well.
- Fill the avocado half shells and sprinkle on some chopped dill to garnish.

Makes 4 appetizer servings or 2 lunch servings.

VARIATION: This salad may also be made with crab meat.

NOTE: Nutrition information is calculated based on 4 servings.

Thanks to our good friend Donna Jones from Nova Scotia for this great recipe.

Nutrition Information per Serving	
Calories	284.01
Protein	12.32 g
Carbs	8.86 g
Fat	24.16 g
Fiber	4.90 g
Net carb	3.96 g

Savory Coleslaw

4 cups finely sliced green cabbage
2 cups finely sliced red cabbage
2 green onions, thinly sliced

Dressing
½ cup real mayonnaise
1 tablespoon lemon juice
1 clove garlic, minced
1 tablespoon white wine vinegar

• Whisk together dressing ingredients until smooth and set aside.
• Cut cabbage and onion into very thin slices and mix in a large bowl with dressing.
• Chill for at least an hour before serving to allow flavors to blend. Will keep up to 48 hours in a fridge.
Makes 8 servings.

TIP: To keep the red color from running, rinse the sliced red cabbage under cold water in a colander, until the water runs clear.

Nutrition Information per Serving

Calories	118.66
Protein	0.94 g
Carbs	3.94 g
Fat	11.17 g
Fiber	1.42 g
Net carb	2.52 g

Spinach Salad

6 cups fresh spinach
2 hard-boiled eggs
4 slices bacon
1 cup sliced raw mushrooms
½ cup roasted almond pieces
1 small sweet red pepper, cut into matchsticks
Red Wine Vinaigrette (see recipe)

• Wash and pat dry the spinach. Cook bacon until crispy and let cool, then chop into pieces. Chop the eggs into small pieces. Combine all ingredients in a large bowl.
• Add the dressing to the salad just before serving.
Makes 4 servings.

Nutrition Information per Serving

Calories	346.92
Protein	11.04 g
Carbs	7.89 g
Fat	31.46 g
Fiber	3.48 g
Net carb	4.41 g

Spinach & Strawberry Salad

6 cups spinach, raw
1 cup sliced strawberries
½ cup toasted almond slivers
¼ cup thinly sliced red onion
Red Wine Vinaigrette (see recipe)

- Toast the almond slivers until lightly browned.
- Wash and pat dry the spinach. Tear off stems and tear leaves into bite-sized pieces.
- Wash and pat dry the strawberries. Slice into thin pieces down the sides to show the shape of the berries.
- Combine all ingredients in a large bowl and toss with Red Wine Vinaigrette.
Makes 4 servings.

Nutrition Information per Serving	
Calories	130.39
Protein	5.60 g
Carbs	8.72 g
Fat	9.50 g
Fiber	4.18 g
Net carb	4.54 g

Summer Salad

5 cups mixed baby greens

1 cup red leaf lettuce

½ medium pear, quartered and thinly sliced

½ cup palm hearts (canned)

1 small avocado, peeled and thinly sliced

To Finish

3 tablespoons chopped fresh flat leaf parsley

Balsamic & Raspberry Vinaigrette (see recipe)

- Prepare all vegetables in a large salad bowl.
- Pour dressing over salad and toss to coat. Sprinkle with fresh parsley.
- Divide evenly among serving plates.

Makes 4 servings.

Nutrition Information per Serving

Calories	272.42
Protein	2.54 g
Carbs	10.30 g
Fat	26.55 g
Fiber	4.03 g
Net carb	6.27 g

Tangy Coleslaw

2 cups finely chopped green cabbage
1 cup finely chopped red cabbage
1 medium carrot, grated
2 green onions, thinly sliced

Dressing
½ cup olive oil
⅓ cup white wine vinegar
1½ teaspoons dry mustard
1 teaspoon ground pepper
1 tablespoon chopped fresh parsley
1 clove garlic, finely minced

• Place the cabbage in a large mixing bowl and add grated carrot and green onion. (I prefer the cabbage to be finely chopped, but you may shred it if you prefer your slaw in very fine pieces.)
• Whisk together all ingredients for the dressing. Pour over cabbage and mix well. Let stand in the fridge for at least an hour before serving.
Makes 6–8 servings.

TIP: To keep the red color from running, rinse the sliced red cabbage under cold water in a colander, until the water runs clear.

NOTE: This coleslaw tastes better the second day, when all the flavors have blended.

Nutrition Information per Serving	
Calories	138.92
Protein	0.49 g
Carbs	2.96 g
Fat	14.13 g
Fiber	0.82 g
Net carb	2.14 g

Tuna Salad

2 cans (6 ounces each) tuna
¼ cup mayonnaise
2 tablespoons lemon juice
1 packet Splenda
1 tablespoon chopped fresh parsley
1 celery stalk, diced
½ cup finely chopped green onion
6 cups red leaf lettuce
2 ripe tomatoes

• Whisk together the mayonnaise, Splenda, lemon juice, and parsley and set aside. Mix together tuna, onion, and celery in a mixing bowl. Fold the dressing with the tuna mixture.

• Evenly distribute the tuna salad over a bed of lettuce. Garnish with tomato wedges.

Makes 4 servings.

Nutrition Information per Serving	
Calories	278.67
Protein	25.16 g
Carbs	2.44 g
Fat	19.13 g
Fiber	0.61 g
Net carb	1.83 g

Waldorf Salad

2 cups cooked, cut-up chicken
2 celery stalks, cut on an angle
½ cup walnut pieces
1 small ripe avocado
6 cups fresh greens
Waldorf Dressing (see recipe)

• Skin and pit the avocado and cut into thin slices. Combine the cut-up chicken, walnuts, and celery in a large mixing bowl. Gently add in the avocado and mix with the dressing.
• Serve on a bed of fresh greens.
Makes 4 servings.

NOTE: This is a delicious alternative to the regular Waldorf salad, with its high-carb apple slivers. To reduce the calories, use only half an avocado in the salad. Also note that much of the fat content comes from the avocado and nuts, which contain the good fats.

Nutrition Information per Serving

Calories	416.67
Protein	18.29 g
Carbs	10.89 g
Fat	34.74 g
Fiber	5.32 g
Net carb	5.57 g

SALAD DRESSINGS & SAUCES

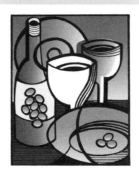

Balsamic Vinaigrette

¼ cup olive oil

⅔ cup balsamic vinegar

1 teaspoon dry mustard

1 teaspoon chopped fresh parsley

1 packet Splenda

½ teaspoon freshly ground pepper

• Whisk together the vinaigrette ingredients.
Makes enough dressing for 4 servings.

Nutrition Information per Serving

Calories	135.57
Protein	0.03 g
Carbs	3.37 g
Fat	14.03 g
Fiber	0.04 g
Net carb	3.33 g

Balsamic & Raspberry Vinaigrette

1½ tablespoons balsamic vinegar
1½ tablespoons raspberry vinegar
1½ tablespoons lemon juice
½ tablespoon chopped fresh flat leaf parsley
⅔ cup olive oil

• Whisk together ingredients for dressing until blended.
Makes enough dressing for 4 servings.

TIP: To make a quick vinaigrette dressing, place all ingredients in a small glass jar. Put the lid on tightly and shake vigorously for 30 seconds to mix.

Nutrition Information per Serving

Calories	168.18
Protein	0.02 g
Carbs	1.62 g
Fat	18.67 g
Fiber	0.02 g
Net carb	1.60 g

Creamy Balsamic Vinaigrette

1 cup balsamic vinegar

3 tablespoons Dijon mustard

4 tablespoons lemon juice

2 tablespoons extra virgin olive oil

2 cloves garlic, minced

1 teaspoon dried thyme leaves (not ground)

1½ teaspoons dried rosemary (not ground)

1 packet Splenda

2 teaspoons chopped fresh parsley

• Put all ingredients in a blender and blend well. You can also use an immersion blender to blend, if desired.

Makes 12 servings of 2 tablespoons each.

Nutrition Information per Serving	
Calories	35.64
Protein	0.46 g
Carbs	2.42 g
Fat	2.71 g
Fiber	0.33 g
Net carb	2.09 g

Creamy Dijon Vinaigrette

¾ cup extra virgin olive oil
⅓ cup red wine vinegar
1 tablespoon Dijon mustard
1 clove garlic, minced
2 teaspoons Worcestershire Sauce
2 packets Splenda
¼ teaspoon ground black pepper
⅛ teaspoon salt

- Put all ingredients in a blender and blend until well combined.
Makes 8 servings of 2 tablespoons each.

Nutrition Information per Serving

Calories	188.54
Protein	0.40 g
Carbs	1.29 g
Fat	21.40 g
Fiber	0.05 g
Net carb	1.24 g

Creamy Raspberry Vinaigrette

½ cup extra virgin olive oil

⅔ cup raspberry vinegar

1 teaspoon Dijon mustard

1 packet Splenda

⅛ teaspoon salt

2 teaspoons chopped fresh parsley

• Put all ingredients in a blender and blend until well combined.
Makes 6 servings of 2 tablespoons each.

**Nutrition Information
per Serving**

Calories	169.17
Protein	0.40 g
Carbs	1.53 g
Fat	19.07 g
Fiber	0.03 g
Net carb	1.50 g

Creamy Vegetable Marinade

juice of 1 lemon

zest of half a lemon

2 tablespoons rice vinegar, unseasoned

½ cup extra virgin olive oil

1 clove garlic, minced

1 tablespoon Dijon mustard

1 packet Splenda

• Blend all marinade ingredients together in a blender.

Makes 4 servings

Nutrition Information per Serving	
Calories	127.46
Protein	0.17 g
Carbs	1.07 g
Fat	14.13 g
Fiber	0.03 g
Net carb	1.04 g

Creamy White Wine Vinaigrette

⅔ cup extra virgin olive oil

3 tablespoons white wine vinegar

1 teaspoon Dijon mustard

1 clove garlic, minced

1 teaspoon dried parsley

1 packet Splenda

¼ teaspoon ground black pepper

⅛ teaspoon salt

- Put all ingredients in a blender and blend until well combined.
Makes 6 servings of 2 tablespoons each.

Nutrition Information per Serving	
Calories	110.08
Protein	0.10 g
Carbs	0.52 g
Fat	12.52 g
Fiber	0.03 g
Net carb	0.49 g

Curried Pineapple Dressing

½ cup mayonnaise

1 tablespoon lemon juice

1 tablespoon unsweetened pineapple juice

½ teaspoon curry powder

1 tablespoon chopped fresh parsley

• Whisk together all ingredients for the dressing.

Makes enough dressing for 4 servings.

Nutrition Information per Serving

Calories	149.27
Protein	0.05 g
Carbs	1.97 g
Fat	16.03 g
Fiber	0.08 g
Net carb	1.89 g

Curried Red Wine Dressing

½ cup light extra virgin olive oil

2 tablespoons lemon juice

2 tablespoons no-sugar-added apricot jam

1 tablespoon red wine vinegar

½ teaspoon curry powder

1 packet Splenda

⅛ teaspoon salt

• This dressing is best if processed with a blender to fully emulsify the jam. *Makes enough dressing for 6 servings.*

Nutrition Information per Serving

Calories	167.77
Protein	0.04 g
Carbs	1.69 g
Fat	18.70 g
Fiber	0.08 g
Net carb	1.61 g

Dijon Vinaigrette

⅔ cup olive oil

4 tablespoons white wine vinegar

2 tablespoons lemon juice

1 teaspoon Dijon mustard

1 teaspoon each chopped fresh rosemary & thyme

2 teaspoons chopped fresh parsley

1 packet Splenda

• Whisk together all ingredients for dressing.
Makes enough dressing for 4 servings.

Nutrition Information per Serving

Calories	170.84
Protein	0.31 g
Carbs	1.85 g
Fat	18.92 g
Fiber	0.08 g
Net carb	1.77 g

Lemon Curry Dressing

½ cup real mayonnaise

2 tablespoons lemon juice

½ teaspoon curry powder

1 tablespoon chopped fresh parsley

• Whisk together all ingredients for the dressing.
Makes enough dressing for 4 servings.

**Nutrition Information
per Serving**

Calories   203.47
Protein   0.06 g
Carbs   0.80 g
Fat   22.03 g
Fiber   0.11 g
Net carb   0.69 g

Oriental Dressing

⅔ cup mayonnaise

4 packets Splenda

2 tablespoons lime juice

2 tablespoons rice vinegar, unseasoned

1 tablespoon soy sauce

½ teaspoon ground ginger

1 teaspoon Sambal Oelek (hot chili sauce)

⅛ teaspoon ground black pepper

• Whisk all dressing ingredients together.
Makes enough dressing for 4 servings.

Nutrition Information per Serving

Calories	75.77
Protein	0.27 g
Carbs	1.38 g
Fat	8.01 g
Fiber	0.03 g
Net carb	1.35 g

Red Wine Vinaigrette

⅔ cup extra virgin olive oil

3 tablespoons red wine vinegar

1 tablespoon lemon juice

1 teaspoon Dijon mustard

1 packet Splenda

¼ teaspoon ground black pepper

⅛ teaspoon salt

- Blend all ingredients in a blender.

Makes enough for 4 servings.

Thanks to Robin Hartzell for the recipe for the dressing; she adapted it from her favorite.

Nutrition Information per Serving	
Calories	168.21
Protein	0.13 g
Carbs	1.33 g
Fat	18.80 g
Fiber	0.06 g
Net carb	1.27 g

Soy Ginger Dressing

¼ cup rice vinegar

3 tablespoons soy sauce

2 teaspoons grated fresh ginger

2 teaspoons toasted sesame oil

1 packet Splenda

• Place all ingredients in a small jar with a tight lid and shake vigorously. Be sure that the ginger is finely grated. Alternatively, blend in a blender to ensure that all ingredients are well blended.
Makes enough for 4 servings.

Nutrition Information per Serving	
Calories	34.85
Protein	0.77 g
Carbs	1.58 g
Fat	2.34 g
Fiber	0.02 g
Net carb	1.56 g

Tangy Red Wine Dressing

⅔ cup olive oil

2 tablespoons red wine vinegar

1 clove garlic, finely minced

1 teaspoon dry mustard

1 packet Splenda

½ teaspoon salt

½ teaspoon freshly ground pepper

• Whisk together all ingredients for the dressing to emulsify.

• Add the dressing to the salad just before serving, if using with spinach salad.

Makes enough dressing for 4 servings.

Nutrition Information per Serving

Calories	169.62
Protein	0.22 g
Carbs	1.25 g
Fat	18.87 g
Fiber	0.09 g
Net carb	1.16 g

Waldorf Dressing

⅔ cup mayonnaise

2 tablespoons heavy cream

1 tablespoon white wine vinegar

1 packet Splenda

¼ teaspoon salt

½ teaspoon freshly ground pepper

- Whisk together all ingredients.

Makes enough dressing for 4 servings.

Nutrition Information per Serving

Calories	161.05
Protein	0.18 g
Carbs	1.52 g
Fat	17.45 g
Fiber	0.03 g
Net carb	1.49 g

White Wine Vinaigrette

⅔ cup olive oil

⅔ cup white wine vinegar

1 teaspoon Dijon mustard

1 teaspoon freshly ground pepper

1 packet Splenda

• Whisk together dressing ingredients.

Makes enough dressing for 6 servings.

Nutrition Information per Serving

Calories	109.41
Protein	0.07 g
Carbs	0.37 g
Fat	12.52 g
Fiber	0.03 g
Net carb	0.34 g

Balsamic Citrus Sauce

2 tablespoons finely minced onion

¼ cup white wine

¼ cup fresh orange juice

1 tablespoon balsamic vinegar

1 teaspoon butter

1 teaspoon orange zest

1 teaspoon each chopped fresh mint & thyme

2 teaspoons chopped fresh parsley

• Place the wine, balsamic vinegar, and orange juice in a small saucepan. Bring to a boil, add the chopped onion, and simmer for 3–4 minutes, until slightly thickened.

• Add the other ingredients and simmer for an additional couple of minutes.

• Serve warm over salmon.

Makes sufficient sauce for 4–6 servings.

Nutrition Information per Serving

Calories	48.36
Protein	0.19 g
Carbs	2.38 g
Fat	2.93 g
Fiber	0.09 g
Net carb	2.29 g

Basil Sauce

½ cup mayonnaise

½ cup fresh basil

2 tablespoons extra virgin olive oil

2 sprigs fresh dill

1 tablespoon chopped chives

1 tablespoon lemon juice

½ tablespoon lemon zest

2 tablespoons chopped fresh parsley

1 green onion, roughly chopped

• Put all the ingredients in a blender and blend until smooth. If you make the sauce beforehand, keep in the fridge until ready to serve.

• Serve with BBQ'd salmon.

Makes enough sauce for 6 servings.

Nutrition Information per Serving	
Calories	193.81
Protein	0.27 g
Carbs	2.12 g
Fat	20.73 g
Fiber	0.34 g
Net carb	1.78 g

BBQ Sauce

2 tablespoons tomato paste

3 tablespoons vegetable oil

1 teaspoon balsamic vinegar

2 teaspoons Worcestershire Sauce

1 teaspoon Kitchen Bouquet

½ teaspoon Mrs. Dash Extra Spicy

½ teaspoon dried thyme

1 teaspoon lime juice

1 teaspoon lemon juice

• Mix all ingredients together with a small whisk. Refrigerate for at least an hour before use.
• Use with ribs, burgers, or chicken.

This makes enough sauce for 4 servings.

Nutrition Information per Serving

Calories	113.64
Protein	1.61 g
Carbs	4.92 g
Fat	11.32 g
Fiber	0.87 g
Net carb	4.05 g

Chocolate Ganache

....

50 grams dark chocolate

⅓ cup heavy cream

- Break up the chocolate in a heat-proof bowl.
- Bring the cream to just below a boil. The cream will steam and begin to ripple when it has reached the proper temperature. Pour the cream over the chocolate and stir vigorously until melted.
- Immediately pour the mix over the cake and let it run down the sides. The chocolate will firm up as it cools.

Makes sufficient ganache to cover a whole cake (10 servings).

NOTE: I like to use Lindt 70% Cocoa Smooth Dark Chocolate bars to make this ganache. Half of the large bar is 50 g. You can use any rich dark chocolate, but the carb content will vary depending on the chocolate that you use.

Nutrition Information per Serving

Calories	54.87
Protein	0.54 g
Carbs	1.85 g
Fat	5.06 g
Fiber	0.25 g
Net carb	1.60 g

Citrus Sauce

3 tablespoons mayonnaise

2 tablespoons fresh orange juice

2 teaspoons fresh lime juice

1 teaspoon fresh lemon juice

1 tablespoon chopped fresh dill weed

½ tablespoon orange zest

- Blend all ingredients with a whisk.
- The orange zest needs to be very fine. Both the zest and the dill add to the flavor and the attractive appearance of this sauce.
- I add the juices a bit at a time until I have the consistency and flavor that I want. It can take a little more or less than the recommended amount, depending on the flavors of your fruits.
- The sauce can be made in advance and kept in the fridge.
- Serve with poached salmon. You want a sauce that pours over the fillets and drips down the sides just a little.

Makes sufficient sauce for 4–6 servings.

Nutrition Information per Serving	
Calories	84.84
Protein	0.04 g
Carbs	1.41 g
Fat	9.01 g
Fiber	0.07 g
Net carb	1.34 g

Cooked Raspberry Purée

1 cup raspberries, either fresh or frozen
6 packets Splenda
1 tablespoon liqueur or sweet dessert wine

• Wash and pat dry raspberries if using fresh fruit. Purée the raspberries in a blender or food processor. You may put them through a sieve if you do not want the seeds in the purée.
• Put the raspberries, Splenda, and liqueur in a small pot and cook over medium heat for 5–10 minutes.
• Cool fully before using as a garnish on any one of many cakes or as an ice-cream topping.

Makes 8 servings of 2 tablespoons each.

NOTE: Nutrition will vary slightly depending on your choice of liqueur.

Nutrition Information per Serving	
Calories	12.09
Protein	0.09 g
Carbs	3.12 g
Fat	0.00 g
Fiber	0.33 g
Net carb	2.79 g

Cranberry Salsa

2 large tangerines
3 cups raw cranberries
½ cup pecan halves
12 packets Splenda

• Place the first tangerine, complete with rind, in a food processor or blender and pulse a couple of times. Add the cranberries, Splenda, and nuts. Peel the second tangerine and add it to the food processor. Process until blended but not puréed.
Makes 16 servings of approximately 2 tablespoons each.

NOTE: This is a great garnish with many dishes but especially served with chicken or white fish.

Thanks to my dad, Greg Tompkins, for this simple and tasty idea.

Nutrition Information per Serving

Calories	41.05
Protein	0.46 g
Carbs	5.01 g
Fat	2.49 g
Fiber	1.43 g
Net carb	3.58 g

Cranberry Sauce

....

1½ cups raw cranberries
¼ cup water
6 packets Splenda
zest of small orange

• Bring all the ingredients to a boil over medium heat. Reduce heat and simmer for 5 minutes.

Makes approximately 1 cup of tart cranberry sauce or 8 servings of 2 tablespoons each.

Nutrition Information per Serving

Calories	8.97
Protein	0.07 g
Carbs	3.07 g
Fat	0.04 g
Fiber	0.77 g
Net carb	2.30 g

Creamy Dill Sauce

⅔ cup mayonnaise
2 teaspoons fresh lemon juice
1 packet Splenda
1 tablespoon chopped fresh dill

- Place all ingredients in a small bowl and whisk until smooth. Keep refrigerated until ready to serve.
- Best if served with cold salmon.

Makes sufficient sauce for 4 servings.

Nutrition Information per Serving

Calories	148.02
Protein	0.03 g
Carbs	2.04 g
Fat	64.00 g
Fiber	0.02 g
Net carb	2.02 g

Creamy Red Wine Sauce

1 cup red wine
½ teaspoon cornstarch
¼ cup beef bouillon
1 teaspoon Dijon mustard
½ teaspoon soy sauce
1 tablespoon chopped fresh parsley
1 teaspoon freshly ground pepper

• Add beef bouillon and cornstarch in a small saucepan and stir to dissolve cornstarch. Add all remaining ingredients and stir to blend well.
• Simmer for 5–6 minutes, stirring constantly, until sauce is thickened. Reduce heat and keep warm until ready to serve.
• Sauce may be poured over meat or served in a serving dish. Serve with roast beef or other red meat.

Makes sufficient sauce for 6–8 servings.

Nutrition Information per Serving	
Calories	34.38
Protein	0.43 g
Carbs	1.83 g
Fat	0.21 g
Fiber	0.12 g
Net carb	1.71 g

Dijon Herb Sauce

1 teaspoon each olive oil & butter

1 clove garlic, finely minced

1 tablespoon finely minced green onion

½ teaspoon dried thyme

½ teaspoon dried rosemary

½ teaspoon Fine Herbs

2 tablespoons Dijon mustard

2 tablespoons grainy Dijon mustard

¼ cup chicken bouillon

• In a small saucepan, over medium-low heat, melt butter and olive oil. Add garlic and onion and sauté 3–4 minutes, until soft. Add the thyme, rosemary, Fine Herbs, and chicken bouillon.

• Bring to a boil and reduce by half, stirring constantly. This will take 4–5 minutes.

• Remove from heat and stir in mustards. Cool and refrigerate until ready to use. May be made the day before and kept in the fridge.

• Best served with rack of lamb.

Makes sufficient sauce for 4–6 servings.

Nutrition Information per Serving	
Calories	37.06
Protein	0.78 g
Carbs	1.96 g
Fat	2.78 g
Fiber	0.30 g
Net carb	1.66 g

Fine Herbs

1 teaspoon dried thyme
1 teaspoon ground savory
1 teaspoon dried oregano
½ teaspoon dried rosemary
¼ teaspoon dried marjoram
¼ teaspoon ground sage
½ teaspoon dried basil
2 teaspoons dried parsley

• Mix all ingredients together well and keep in an airtight container.
Makes 13 servings of 1/2 teaspoon each.

TIP: I prefer to use the whole dried spices in this blend rather than the ground spices. Doing so adds both texture and flavor.

NOTE: I have included this recipe for a French spice blend because manufacturers no longer seem to be making this mix called Fines Herbes. In some cases, the mixture of herbs is changing and does not taste the same. I use this spice a lot, so I have experimented with various options, and this is the blend that I like the best. I have recently found a new spice blend called Herbes de Provence, a French blend with a slightly different flavor that can be used instead of Fines Herbes.

Nutrition Information per Serving	
Calories	2.58
Protein	0.06 g
Carbs	0.30 g
Fat	0.03 g
Fiber	0.14 g
Net carb	0.16 g

Fresh Herb Salsa

½ bunch of fresh flat leaf parsley (regular fresh parsley will do)
10 fresh basil leaves
10 fresh mint leaves
1 clove garlic, minced
1 tablespoon Dijon mustard
1 teaspoon red wine vinegar
⅔ cup olive oil
salt & freshly ground pepper, to taste

• Finely chop all the herbs. Add vinegar, oil, and garlic and mix in blender or food processor to emulsify.
• Add salt & pepper to taste and let stand at room temperature in a covered dish for 30 minutes to blend flavors.
Makes sufficient salsa for 4–6 servings.

Nutrition Information per Serving	
Calories	165.09
Protein	0.91 g
Carbs	1.28 g
Fat	19.26 g
Fiber	0.16 g
Net carb	1.12 g

Hollandaise Sauce

2 egg yolks
6 teaspoons butter
3 teaspoons lemon juice
⅛ teaspoon salt

- Place egg yolks and 2 teaspoons of butter in the top of a double boiler, over simmering water. Stir constantly with a whisk until butter melts.
- Add 2 teaspoons of butter and continue cooking. The sauce may start to thicken as you add the final 2 teaspoons of butter. Continue to cook and whisk until the butter is completely melted.
- Remove top of double boiler to a tea towel (to absorb any extra moisture) on nearby counter. Continue to whisk for 2 minutes. Add 3 teaspoons of lemon juice in 3 equal portions while whisking continuously.
- Add the salt and put back on top of double boiler for 2–3 minutes, until thickened, stirring constantly.
- If the sauce thickens too much, or starts to curdle, add 1–2 tablespoons of boiling water.

Makes approximately ½ cup of Hollandaise Sauce.

NOTE: This will make just enough for two servings of eggs Benedict that are not drowned in the sauce. The recipe may be doubled if you like lots of sauce.

Nutrition Information per Serving

Calories	162.84
Protein	2.93 g
Carbs	0.80 g
Fat	16.66 g
Fiber	0.03 g
Net carb	0.77 g

Lemon Herb Marinade for Chicken

¼ cup olive oil
2 tablespoons lemon juice
1 teaspoon Fine Herbs
1 teaspoon dried thyme
1 teaspoon dried rosemary
pinch of salt
freshly ground pepper, to taste

- Whisk together ingredients for marinade.
Makes sufficient marinade for 4–6 chicken breasts.

Nutrition Information per Serving

Calories	128.07
Protein	0.24 g
Carbs	1.41 g
Fat	14.15 g
Fiber	0.31 g
Net carb	1.10 g

Lemon Herb Marinade for Pork

zest and juice of 1 medium lemon

2 tablespoons white wine

1 tablespoon olive oil

2 garlic cloves, minced

1 tablespoon each chopped fresh thyme, parsley, & mint

1 teaspoon freshly ground pepper

½ teaspoon salt

- In a small bowl, whisk together all ingredients.
- Pour over pork and let sit in the fridge for at least an hour.

Makes sufficient marinade for 4–6 servings.

Nutrition Information per Serving

Calories	44.66
Protein	0.29 g
Carbs	2.29 g
Fat	3.58 g
Fiber	0.36 g
Net carb	1.93 g

Lemon Thyme Marinade for Chicken

¼ cup lemon juice

1 tablespoon chopped fresh thyme

½ tablespoon chopped fresh rosemary

1 tablespoon Dijon mustard

1 teaspoon freshly ground pepper

½ teaspoon salt

- Whisk together all ingredients and let sit for a few minutes to blend flavors.
- Pour over chicken and let sit in the fridge for about an hour.

Makes sufficient marinade for 4–6 servings.

Nutrition Information per Serving	
Calories	11.20
Protein	0.44 g
Carbs	2.21 g
Fat	0.31 g
Fiber	0.34 g
Net carb	1.87 g

Lemon Thyme Sauce

1 tablespoon butter
juice of 1 lemon
1 teaspoon lemon zest
1 tablespoon each chopped fresh thyme & parsley
½ tablespoon chopped fresh rosemary
½ cup heavy cream
1 teaspoon cornstarch
½ teaspoon salt

• Melt butter over medium heat in a small saucepan. Add herbs and sauté for 2 minutes, stirring constantly. Add the juice and zest of the lemon.
• Gradually add the heavy cream and cornstarch. (Dissolve cornstarch in a small amount of water before adding to the sauce.) Add the salt.
• Simmer for 5–6 minutes, stirring constantly, until the sauce thickens.
• Serve warm from a gravy dish or other serving dish. Best if served with salmon.
Makes 4–6 servings.

NOTE: If the sauce is a bit tart, add additional salt, to taste, to diminish the tartness. The tartness varies with the size and flavor of each lemon. This sauce may be made 2–3 hours ahead of time, kept in the fridge, and reheated gently over a low element.

Nutrition Information per Serving	
Calories	90.51
Protein	0.52 g
Carbs	1.98 g
Fat	9.32 g
Fiber	0.16 g
Net carb	1.82 g

Mustard Dipping Sauce

2 tablespoons Dijon mustard
1 teaspoon mayonnaise
2 packets Splenda
1 teaspoon white wine vinegar

- Whisk together all the ingredients until smooth.
- Serve in small dishes for dipping. This sauce may be served with chicken tenders or spicy chicken wings.

Makes sufficient dipping sauce for 4 servings.

Nutrition Information per Serving

Calories	12.28
Protein	1.00 g
Carbs	1.37 g
Fat	1.61 g
Fiber	0.00 g
Net carb	1.37 g

Orange Marinade

¼ cup fresh orange juice (juice of small orange)
1 tablespoon orange zest
2 tablespoons olive oil
4 teaspoons soy sauce

• Whisk together the ingredients and pour over chicken breasts. Let the chicken sit in the fridge for at least an hour.
Makes sufficient marinade for 4–6 breasts.

Thanks to my friend Sarah Smith for sharing the basic ingredients of this great marinade.

Nutrition Information per Serving	
Calories	73.67
Protein	0.87 g
Carbs	2.32 g
Fat	7.12 g
Fiber	0.10 g
Net carb	2.22 g

Oriental Stir-Fry Sauce

3 tablespoons tomato paste
3 tablespoons soy sauce
1 teaspoon toasted sesame oil
2 cloves garlic, minced
1 packet Splenda
2 tablespoons grated fresh ginger
1 teaspoon sesame seeds, to garnish

• Finely grate the fresh ginger. Add the remaining ingredients except the sesame seeds. Whisk all ingredients to blend well.
• Add the sauce to the dish just before finishing. Mix well and continue cooking for 3–4 minutes to ensure that the sauce is hot and well distributed.
• Sprinkle sesame seeds on top of finished dish to garnish.
Makes 4 servings.

NOTE: This sauce may be used as a stir fry sauce for any oriental-style dish.

Thanks to Lisa Shaw of Victoria, British Columbia, for this really simple and delicious sauce.

Nutrition Information per Serving

Calories	31.88
Protein	1.35 g
Carbs	4.32 g
Fat	1.26 g
Fiber	0.60 g
Net carb	3.72 g

Raspberry Purée

••

½ cup fresh or frozen unsweetened raspberries
2 packets Splenda

• Thaw berries if frozen. Wash and pat dry berries if using fresh fruit.
• Blend berries with Splenda in a food processor until smooth. You may sift the purée if you do not like the seeds.
• This is a wonderful garnish with fresh fruit, chocolate cakes, and other desserts. It can be drizzled over the dish or used as a base sauce covering a plate before placing the dessert on the plate.
Makes 6 servings.

Nutrition Information per Serving	
Calories	4.17
Protein	0.04 g
Carbs	1.25 g
Fat	0.00 g
Fiber	0.17 g
Net carb	1.08 g

Red Wine Steak Sauce

2 tablespoons butter
½ cup chopped green onion
1 packet Splenda
2 cloves garlic, minced
1 tablespoon fresh rosemary, chopped
1 tablespoon fresh thyme, chopped
1½ cups beef bouillon
¼ cup red wine
2 teaspoons cornstarch

• This sauce is made in a saucepan on the stove. Heat the butter over medium heat and add the onion. Sauté for approximately 5 minutes, until soft.
• Stir in Splenda and herbs and continue cooking for another minute.
• Add beef bouillon and wine and bring the mixture to a boil. Simmer for about 10 minutes until the sauce is reduced by half.
• Add the cornstarch to a little water to dissolve it and then add it to the wine sauce. Stir well to blend and cook for another 5 minutes.
Makes sufficient sauce for 4–6 servings.

NOTE: You can make this sauce in the time it takes to cook your steak. May be drizzled over the steak, served on the plate on the side, or served in a small gravy dish.

Nutrition Information per Serving

Calories	40.39
Protein	0.33 g
Carbs	1.85 g
Fat	2.93 g
Fiber	0.24 g
Net carb	1.61 g

Spicy BBQ Sauce

2 tablespoons tomato paste
3 tablespoons vegetable oil
2 teaspoons Worcestershire Sauce
1 teaspoon Kitchen Bouquet
½ teaspoon Mrs. Dash Extra Spicy
1 teaspoon dried thyme
1 teaspoon dried rosemary
1 teaspoon cayenne
2 teaspoons lime juice
1 teaspoon lemon juice

• Mix all the ingredients together with a small whisk. Refrigerate for at least an hour before use.
• Use with ribs, chicken, or meat.
This makes enough sauce for 4 servings.

Nutrition Information per Serving	
Calories	117.14
Protein	1.69 g
Carbs	5.64 g
Fat	11.40 g
Fiber	1.05 g
Net carb	4.59 g

Vanilla Custard Sauce

1 cup milk
½ cup heavy cream
1 long vanilla bean (6")
4 egg yolks
10 packets Splenda
1 teaspoon cornstarch

• Combine milk, cream, and vanilla bean in a heavy saucepan. Place the saucepan over medium heat and bring the liquid just to a boil.
• Remove from heat and let stand for 10 minutes to absorb the vanilla flavor. Stir occasionally while cooling.
• In a mixing bowl, whisk the egg yolks until smooth. Gradually add the Splenda and continue whisking until the mixture is paler yellow and creamy — about 3 minutes. Add in the cornstarch and whisk well to blend. Stir the milk mixture into the yolks, whisking vigorously.
• Return this mixture to the saucepan and cook over low heat, stirring constantly, until the mixture is quite thick and coats the back of a wooden spoon. This will take 10–15 minutes. Do not let the custard boil at this point.
• Remove from heat and let cool, stirring frequently. Remove the vanilla bean, cover the custard, and chill.
• Serve as a sauce to be poured over individual servings of almond carrot cake.
Makes 12 servings of 3 tablespoons each.

NOTE: This is a really delicious vanilla custard sauce. It can be used warm or chilled over fruit or any low-carb cake.

Nutrition Information per Serving	
Calories	70.69
Protein	1.80 g
Carbs	2.32 g
Fat	6.05 g
Fiber	0.01 g
Net carb	2.31 g

Warm Chocolate Sauce

⅔ cup and 1½ tablespoons heavy cream
1 tablespoon butter
½ teaspoon vanilla extract
100 grams Lindt 70% Cocoa Dark Chocolate

• Melt butter over medium heat in a small saucepan. Add cream and stir to combine while heating until hot (but not boiling).
• Remove from heat and add roughly chopped chocolate. Stir vigorously until chocolate is melted.
• Add the vanilla.
• For a slightly thinner sauce, increase the amount of cream.
• Use immediately as a sauce over low-carb cakes, low-carb ice cream, or fresh fruit. Or store at room temperature in an airtight container and reheat slowly to use at another time. If the chocolate and butter separate when reheating, use a little extra hot cream to help emulsify.

Makes 8 servings of 2 tablespoons each.

Nutrition Information per Serving

Calories	126.14
Protein	1.21 g
Carbs	4.45 g
Fat	11.46 g
Fiber	0.63 g
Net carb	3.82 g

Whipped Cream

½ cup heavy cream
2 packets Splenda

- Beat the heavy cream with the Splenda, until stiff peaks form.
- Use as a nice creamy garnish with sugar-free Jell-O or with fresh fruit or other desserts.

Makes 4–6 servings.

Nutrition Information per Serving

Calories	68.42
Protein	0.41 g
Carbs	0.89 g
Fat	7.34 g
Fiber	0.00 g
Net carb	0.89 g

White Sauce

....

6 teaspoons butter
2 tablespoons flour
2½ cups light cream (half & half)
½ teaspoon salt
1 teaspoon freshly ground pepper
1 tablespoon chopped fresh parsley

• In the top of a double boiler, over simmering water, melt butter and add
flour. Stir until smooth and completely blended.
• Gradually add the light cream, stirring constantly to avoid any lumps. Add
the salt, pepper, and parsley.
• Cook over the simmering water until the white sauce has thickened, about 15
minutes, stirring almost constantly to avoid any lumps.
Makes 8 servings of approximately ¼ cup each.

**Nutrition Information
per Serving**

Calories	178.12
Protein	2.29 g
Carbs	4.07 g
Fat	17.40 g
Fiber	0.02 g
Net carb	4.05 g

VEGETABLES

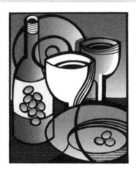

Asparagus in Foil

1 pound fresh asparagus
2 tablespoons lemon juice
4 tablespoons extra virgin olive oil
1 clove garlic, minced
1 tablespoon chopped fresh parsley
salt & pepper, to taste

• Wash and pat dry the asparagus spears. Place in a shallow dish.
• Whisk together the olive oil, lemon juice, minced garlic, parsley, and salt & pepper. Pour over asparagus and marinate for an hour, turning occasionally.
• Place asparagus in the center of a large piece of tin foil and tent, being sure to seal all the seams.
• Place on a BBQ that has been preheated to a medium-high temperature. Cook for 10 minutes. Carefully open the foil wrap to let steam escape.
Makes 4 servings.

VARIATION: Place the foil bag on a cookie sheet and cook in an oven at 400° for 10 minutes.

Nutrition Information per Serving

Calories	149.14
Protein	2.69 g
Carbs	5.95 g
Fat	14.26 g
Fiber	2.46 g
Net carb	3.49 g

Asparagus with Balsamic Vinegar

1 pound asparagus

1 tablespoon olive oil

2 garlic cloves, minced

2 tablespoons butter

4 tablespoons balsamic vinegar

4 tablespoons water

1 tablespoon chopped fresh parsley

1 teaspoon freshly ground pepper

• Heat oil in a nonstick frying pan over medium heat. Add garlic and parsley and cook for 2 minutes, stirring constantly. Add balsamic vinegar, water, and butter to the pan and cook until blended, about 1 minute.

• Add the asparagus and pepper to the pan and simmer until tender, approximately 5 minutes.

• Place asparagus on plates.

Makes 4 servings.

Nutrition Information per Serving	
Calories	113.67
Protein	2.70 g
Carbs	5.87 g
Fat	9.50 g
Fiber	2.44 g
Net carb	3.43 g

Broccoli Soufflé

4 eggs, separated

1 cup broccoli florets

½ cup shredded cheddar cheese

1 cup light cream (half & half)

1 tablespoon flour

½ teaspoon salt

1 tablespoon sour cream

1 teaspoon heavy cream

- Preheat oven to 300°.
- Steam florets for 10 minutes or until soft. Put florets in a food processor with sour cream and heavy cream and purée. Set aside. You will have about ½ cup of the purée.
- In the top of a double boiler, over boiling water, heat light cream for 2–3 minutes. Whisk in flour until smooth and thickened, about 3 minutes. Add shredded cheese and whisk until completely blended, about 5 minutes. Remove from heat.
- In a large separate bowl, beat egg whites until very stiff. Add egg yolks to the cheese mixture, one at a time, whisking after each addition. Fold in the puréed broccoli to the cheese mixture.
- Gradually, working in 4–5 batches, fold the cheese and broccoli mixture into the egg white.
- Pour into an ungreased, 1½-quart casserole dish, until ¼″ from the top.
- Place casserole in the center of the oven and bake for 60 minutes. Do not open oven door while soufflé is baking. Serve at once.

Makes 4 servings.

VARIATION: For a two-cheese soufflé, cut out the broccoli purée and substitute a 1/2 cup of another shredded cheese, such as Swiss cheese.

NOTE: This makes a lovely lunch with a small green salad. It is also a nice vegetable as an accompaniment to a chicken dish.

Nutrition Information per Serving

Calories	237.40
Protein	13.32 g
Carbs	6.66 g
Fat	17.82 g
Fiber	0.66 g
Net carb	6.00 g

Broccoli Supreme

¾ pound broccoli florets
2 cups chicken bouillon
1 tablespoon butter
½ medium sweet onion, diced
1 tablespoon chopped fresh
  parsley
½ tablespoon each chopped
  fresh chives & thyme

⅓ cup sour cream
¼ cup heavy cream
½ teaspoon freshly ground
  pepper
salt, to taste
chopped fresh parsley, to
  garnish

• Bring the chicken bouillon to a boil and add the florets. Cover and simmer until the florets are soft, about 15 minutes.
• While the broccoli is simmering, in a small saucepan, melt butter over medium heat. Sauté onions until soft, about 4 minutes. Add fresh herbs and sauté for a minute longer. Remove from heat and set aside.
• Drain the broccoli and place it in a food processor with the onion and herb mixture as well as the sour cream and heavy cream. Process until smooth.
• The broccoli may be refrigerated at this point or frozen when cooled and then reheated when ready to serve. If serving right away, return to the stove over low heat to keep warm. Garnish with chopped fresh parsley.
Makes 4 servings.

NOTE: This is a very tasty side dish that is a rich dark green and looks wonderful on the plate.

Special thanks to my friend Pearl Rudin for the idea for this dish.

Nutrition Information per Serving	
Calories	124.24
Protein	0.71 g
Carbs	3.37 g
Fat	12.44 g
Fiber	0.33 g
Net carb	3.04 g

Creaded Spinach

10 cups raw spinach
2 tablespoons butter
1 teaspoon cornstarch
¼ cup heavy cream
¼ cup light cream
½ teaspoon ground black pepper

• Wash and pat dry the spinach. Place in a large saucepan with just a ¼ cup of water. Bring to a boil, reduce heat, and simmer for 3–4 minutes, turning constantly with a fork to ensure that all the spinach is cooked.

• Remove from the heat. Do not drain. Add butter and stir to melt and distribute evenly.

• Dissolve the cornstarch in the two creams. Add to the spinach and return to the heat. Cook, stirring constantly until the cream sauce has thickened, about 5 minutes.

• Serve in small side dishes.

Makes 4 servings.

Nutrition Information per Serving	
Calories	153.43
Protein	2.94 g
Carbs	4.91 g
Fat	14.44 g
Fiber	2.05 g
Net carb	2.86 g

Creamy Cauliflower with Rosemary

1 cauliflower, approximately 1½ pounds
1 tablespoon butter
1 tablespoon olive oil
3 small green onions, chopped
1 tablespoon fresh rosemary, roughly chopped
½ cup whole milk
½ teaspoon ground black pepper
¼ teaspoon salt
½ teaspoon cornstarch
¼ cup heavy cream
¼ cup shredded white cheddar cheese

• Roughly chop the head of cauliflower into 6–8 sections.
• Heat olive oil and butter in a large saucepan over medium heat. Add the chopped green onion and sauté for 2–3 minutes.
• Add the milk, cauliflower, and chopped rosemary. Bring the milk to a boil and reduce heat. Cover and simmer the cauliflower until done, about 15 minutes.
• Break the cauliflower into bite-sized pieces using a fork. Dissolve the cornstarch in the heavy cream and add to the cauliflower. Stir to distribute evenly and continue to cook for another 3 or 4 minutes, until thickened.
• Serve the cauliflower with a sprinkle of white cheddar cheese on top.
Makes 6 servings.

Nutrition Information per Serving	
Calories	134.33
Protein	4.33 g
Carbs	7.80 g
Fat	10.45 g
Fiber	2.94 g
Net carb	4.86 g

Creamy Garlic Cauliflower

1 medium cauliflower (about 4 cups of florets)
1 medium onion, minced
2 cups chicken bouillon
2 garlic cloves, minced
2 teaspoons butter
¼ cup sour cream
¼ cup heavy cream
1 tablespoon chopped fresh chives or parsley

• Wash cauliflower and cut into small florets.
• Bring chicken bouillon to a boil in a large saucepan and add cauliflower. Simmer until soft, about 15 minutes.
• While cauliflower is simmering, sauté onion and garlic in 1 teaspoon of butter in a small saucepan over medium heat. Cook until soft, about 3–4 minutes.
• Drain cauliflower when soft. Add cauliflower, onion, and garlic as well as sour cream, heavy cream, and an additional teaspoon of butter to a food processor and process until smooth. You may have to process in batches, depending on the size of your processor.
• At this point, the cauliflower may be refrigerated or frozen until ready to use. If using immediately, reheat gently in original saucepan. Serve sprinkled with chopped chives or parsley. *Makes 6 servings.*

TIP: This is a great substitute for mashed potatoes, and I often serve it with meat loaf, for just this reason.

Nutrition Information per Serving	
Calories	82.05
Protein	1.22 g
Carbs	3.51 g
Fat	7.12 g
Fiber	0.47 g
Net carb	3.04 g

Creamy Zucchini

2 medium zucchini with skin
3 green onions
1 tablespoon butter
2 cloves garlic, minced
½ tablespoon Dijon mustard
1 cup chicken broth
1 teaspoon dried thyme (not ground)

1 teaspoon Fine Herbs
¼ teaspoon salt
½ teaspoon ground black pepper
1 tablespoon cornstarch
¼ cup sour cream

• Grate zucchini (with skin on) using large holes of grater over paper towel. You should have approximately 6 cups. Squeeze the zucchini to remove most of the moisture.
• Thinly slice the green onions.
• Melt butter over medium heat in a large saucepan. Whisk in the mustard and chicken broth, increase heat, and bring to a boil. Boil uncovered, stirring occasionally, until the liquid is reduced by half. This will take about 5 minutes.
• Add zucchini, onions, thyme, Fine Herbs, and salt & pepper. Cook, stirring often until tender, about 4 minutes.
• In a small dish, add some liquid from the pot to the cornstarch to dissolve. Add this mixture back into the pot and continue to boil, stirring constantly until the mixture is thickened. This will take an additional 2–3 minutes.
• Remove from heat and stir in the sour cream.
Makes 6 servings.

Nutrition Information per Serving	
Calories	66.71
Protein	1.29 g
Carbs	4.69 g
Fat	4.92 g
Fiber	1.02 g
Net carb	3.67 g

Crowned Cauliflower

1 medium whole cauliflower
1 cup grated cheddar cheese
¼ cup mayonnaise
2 teaspoons Dijon mustard
½ teaspoon cayenne pepper
½ teaspoon salt

• Wash the cauliflower and remove all leaves and the woody stem. Place the cauliflower on a pie plate with a ½″ of water. Cover and microwave until cooked. This will take approximately 10–12 minutes.
• While the cauliflower is cooking, turn on the broiler. Then grate the cheese and mix it with the mayonnaise, mustard, cayenne, and salt to make a paste.
• Remove the cauliflower from the microwave and transfer it to a broiling pan. Cover the top and sides of the cauliflower with the cheese topping (crown the cauliflower!). Grill until the cheese melts and starts to brown.
• To serve the crowned cauliflower, cut it into sections. This is a delicious new way to prepare cauliflower.
Makes 6–8 portions depending on the size of the cauliflower.

TIP: Leftover cauliflower can be refrigerated and reheated the next day.

Thanks to Pat Smith of Red Deer, Alberta, for sharing this with us. Pat suggests adding some of the leftover vegetable to eggs for a yummy omelet in the morning.

Nutrition Information per Serving

Calories	130.98
Protein	4.78 g
Carbs	2.25 g
Fat	11.73 g
Fiber	0.89 g
Net carb	1.36 g

Dijon Cabbage with Pecans

4 cups cabbage, chopped
1 cup roughly grated carrot
½ cup thinly sliced red onion
1 cup chicken boullion
2 tablespoons butter
½ cup pecans, chopped
2 tablespoons Dijon mustard
½ teaspoon paprika
¼ teaspoon salt
½ teaspoon ground black pepper

• Bring broth to a boil in a large saucepan. Add cabbage, carrot, onion, and salt & pepper.
• Toss ingredients to mix well and cook, covered, for about 5 minutes until tender. Stir occasionally.
• Combine butter, Dijon mustard, and pecans. Pour over vegetables and toss again. Sprinkle with paprika.
Makes 6 servings.

Nutrition Information per Serving

Calories	136.42
Protein	2.49 g
Carbs	8.06 g
Fat	11.59 g
Fiber	3.20 g
Net carb	4.86 g

Garlic Cauliflower with Pine Nuts

1½–2 pounds cauliflower
2 teaspoons fresh lemon juice
⅓ cup olive oil
1 teaspoon paprika
2 cups water
½ teaspoon salt
1 teaspoon freshly ground pepper
2 garlic cloves, minced
½ cup pine nuts, coarsely chopped
2 tablespoons chopped fresh parsley

• An hour before serving, fill a large bowl with water and add the lemon juice. Wash the cauliflower and cut it into florets. Place cauliflower in the liquid and set aside.
• About 20 minutes before serving, heat the olive oil in a large nonstick frying pan over medium heat. Add the paprika and garlic and cook for 1–2 minutes. Add the 2 cups of water and bring to a boil.
• Drain the cauliflower from the cold water and add to the boiling water in the pan. Season with salt and cook uncovered until cauliflower is tender, approximately 15 minutes.
• Add the chopped nuts and fresh parsley. Season with salt & pepper and continue cooking for 2 minutes. The liquid evaporates while cooking.
• Serve on individual plates.
Makes 6 servings.

Nutrition Information per Serving

Calories	181.74
Protein	4.49 g
Carbs	9.48 g
Fat	15.68 g
Fiber	4.14 g
Net carb	5.34 g

Green Beans
with Bacon & Mushrooms

1 pound fresh green beans
1 teaspoon olive oil
½ cup finely diced fresh mushrooms
4 slices bacon chopped into ¼″ slices
2 green onions cut into ¼″ pieces
freshly ground pepper, to taste

To Finish
¼ cup heavy cream
chopped fresh parsley, to garnish

• Clean and trim beans to desired size. Steam beans until just tender, about 4–6 minutes. Pat dry on a paper towel and put to one side.
• Heat olive oil in a large frying pan or saucepan over medium heat. Sauté bacon, mushrooms, and onion until cooked, about 3–5 minutes. Stir in beans and season with pepper. Add cream and heat through while stirring constantly, about 2–3 minutes.
• Transfer to serving platter or individual plates and garnish with chopped parsley.
Makes 4 servings.

**Nutrition Information
per Serving**

Calories	91.14
Protein	4.94 g
Carbs	9.26 g
Fat	4.41 g
Fiber	4.08 g
Net carb	5.18 g

Green Beans in Curry

1 pound fresh green beans
1 can (14 ounces) coconut milk
¼ cup minced onion
1 clove garlic, finely minced
1 teaspoon curry powder
½ teaspoon cumin
½ teaspoon olive oil

• Heat oil in a heavy frying pan over medium-high heat. Sauté garlic and onion for 2–3 minutes, until soft. Although this is a small amount of oil, the onions will sweat and release moisture as they cook. Add coconut milk and spices and bring mixture to a boil.
• Add trimmed green beans to the milk, cover, and simmer for 10 minutes.
Makes 6 servings.

Nutrition Information per Serving

Calories	162.02
Protein	2.90 g
Carbs	8.27 g
Fat	14.69 g
Fiber	2.77 g
Net carb	5.50 g

Green Beans with Mustard

¾ pound green beans
2 teaspoons olive oil
1½ teaspoons Dijon mustard
2 garlic cloves, finely minced

• Clean and trim beans. Add beans to a pot of boiling water and cook for just 2–3 minutes, until tender crisp. Drain beans and set aside in a container.
• Heat oil in a large nonstick frying pan over medium heat. Add garlic and mustard and stir for 1 minute. Add beans and continue cooking, while stirring, for another 4–5 minutes.
Makes 4 servings.

Nutrition Information per Serving

Calories	25.20
Protein	0.54 g
Carbs	1.13 g
Fat	2.72 g
Fiber	0.20 g
Net carb	0.93 g

Green Beans
with Onions & Vinegar

1 pound green beans
1 medium red onion, thinly sliced
1 teaspoon freshly ground pepper
2 tablespoons olive oil
3 tablespoons red wine vinegar
1 teaspoon Dijon mustard

• Clean and trim the green beans. Bring 2 cups of water to boil in a large saucepan. Add beans and cook until just tender crisp, about 3–4 minutes. Drain and set aside briefly.
• In a large frying pan, heat oil over medium-high heat. Sauté onion for 3–4 minutes and then add beans. Whisk together mustard and red wine vinegar. Add to the pan and stir well while continuing to cook for 2 minutes.
Makes 4 servings.

Nutrition Information per Serving

Calories	38.40
Protein	0.70 g
Carbs	3.58 g
Fat	2.64 g
Fiber	0.74 g
Net carb	2.84 g

Green Beans with Tomato

1 pound green beans
1 tablespoon butter
1 clove garlic, minced
3 small ripe tomatoes, roughly chopped
2 tablespoons chicken broth
1 tablespoon chopped fresh parsley
½ teaspoon freshly ground pepper
¼ teaspoon salt

• Melt butter over medium heat in a large frying pan and add garlic, salt & pepper, and parsley. Cook for just 1 minute, until fragrant.
• Add the green beans, chopped tomato, and chicken stock and stir well. Cover and cook, stirring occasionally, until beans are tender. This will take approximately 10 minutes.
Makes 4 servings.

Nutrition Information per Serving

Calories	74.69
Protein	2.80 g
Carbs	11.13 g
Fat	3.17 g
Fiber	4.52 g
Net carb	6.61 g

Grilled Asparagus with Lemon Butter

1 pound fresh asparagus
2 tablespoons butter
1 teaspoon fresh lemon juice
1 teaspoon chopped fresh parsley
2 tablespoons olive oil
3 teaspoons fresh lemon juice
1 tablespoon chopped fresh mint
1 garlic clove, finely minced

• At least an hour before serving, bring butter to room temperature. Add 1 teaspoon each of the lemon juice and fresh parsley and mix well. Swirl into small rounds and place on waxed paper. Place in the fridge to harden.
• Wash and trim the ends of the asparagus. Using wooden skewers that have been soaked in water for at least an hour, thread two parallel skewers through 4 asparagus. Alternatively, use a grilling basket or rack to grill the asparagus.
• Whisk together the olive oil, mint, garlic, and lemon juice.
• Place the skewered asparagus on a shallow serving plate and pour over the olive oil mixture. Turn to coat and let sit for 30 minutes at room temperature.
• Preheat the BBQ to medium. Brush the asparagus with any remaining marinade and place on the grill. Brush remaining liquid on the upside. Turn asparagus after 2–3 minutes and grill for an additional 2–3 minutes. Do not leave the grill since these delicious vegetables can burn very easily.

continued

• Remove from the grill and slide off the skewers. Place on plates and put a patty of lemon butter on each bunch of asparagus.
Makes 4 servings.

TIP: For grilling, you will want to choose large asparagus, unlike when you are steaming them and looking for the smaller ones. The asparagus can be grilled without being skewered, but skewering makes them easier to handle. The lemon butter can be used on many different vegetables and fish.

Nutrition Information per Serving

Calories	138.50
Protein	2.72 g
Carbs	5.48 g
Fat	13.00 g
Fiber	2.44 g
Net carb	3.04 g

Grilled Eggplant

1 medium eggplant
1½–2 tablespoons light olive oil
2 teaspoons lemon juice
1 tablespoon chopped fresh parsley
1 tablespoon freshly ground pepper

- Preheat the BBQ or grill to medium heat.
- Mix the lemon juice, parsley, and pepper with the olive oil.
- Slice the eggplant into slices between ¼″ and ½″ thick. Brush both sides of the eggplant with the olive oil mixture.
- Place the slices on the grill for 2–3 minutes a side, until golden brown grill marks appear and they are cooked through.

Makes 4–6 servings of 2 slices per serving, depending on the size of the eggplant.

NOTE: Nutrition information is calculated based on 4 servings.

Nutrition Information per Serving	
Calories	80.96
Protein	1.43 g
Carbs	8.38 g
Fat	5.50 g
Fiber	3.46 g
Net carb	4.92 g

Grilled Zucchini

2 medium zucchini
2 tablespoons olive oil
¼ teaspoon paprika
½ teaspoon dried parsley
½ teaspoon dried thyme
1 teaspoon freshly ground pepper

- Preheat grill to medium high.
- Add spices to olive oil in a small dish.
- Cut zucchini in half lengthwise. Brush both sides of zucchini with olive oil mixture.
- Place zucchini on grill, cut side down. Grill for 2–3 minutes a side, depending on the thickness. Test with a fork to determine doneness.
Makes 4 servings.

VARIATION: You may slice the zucchini into 1/2″ rounds, which will grill more quickly.

Nutrition Information per Serving	
Calories	81.94
Protein	1.23 g
Carbs	3.42 g
Fat	7.22 g
Fiber	1.33 g
Net carb	2.09 g

Lemon Cabbage

2 tablespoons olive oil
1 medium head green cabbage
juice of one lemon
1 tablespoon lemon zest
1 cup fresh snow peas, washed and trimmed
1 cup chicken bouillon
salt & freshly ground pepper, to taste

• Wash cabbage and slice thinly into bite-sized pieces.
• Heat olive oil in a large frying pan. Add cabbage and sprinkle with lemon juice and zest. Add salt & pepper, to taste.
• Cook, stirring constantly, for 2–3 minutes. Mix in trimmed snow peas. Simmer gently, stirring occasionally, for 5–6 minutes, until cabbage is tender but crisp.
• Serve using slotted spoon to drain.
Makes 4 servings.

TIP: The snow peas add color and carbohydrates. To reduce the carbohydrates, reduce the amount of snow peas.

Nutrition Information per Serving

Calories	109.00
Protein	4.37 g
Carbs	7.13 g
Fat	11.40 g
Fiber	0.17 g
Net carb	6.96 g

Puréed Turnip & Carrots

2 cups cubed turnip
1½ cups sliced carrot
1 tablespoon butter
1 packet Splenda
¼ teaspoon cinnamon

• Bring the sliced carrots and cubed turnip to a boil in a large saucepan. Boil until tender, approximately 15 minutes.
• Remove from heat and drain. Place the cooked vegetables in a food processor or blender with the butter, Splenda, and cinnamon. Process to the desired smoothness. Add salt & pepper, to taste.
Makes 4 servings.

Nutrition Information per Serving

Calories	69.68
Protein	1.26 g
Carbs	10.55 g
Fat	3.05 g
Fiber	3.18 g
Net carb	7.37 g

Red Cabbage Casserole

1 small turnip (about 1 pound)
1 head red cabbage (about 1½ pounds)
1 medium sweet onion, thinly sliced
¼ cup toasted almond slivers
1 packet Splenda
1½ cups chicken bouillon
½ cup white wine
salt & freshly ground pepper, to taste

- Preheat oven to 350°.
- Wash, trim, and thinly slice the cabbage. Julienne the turnip and place all vegetables and almond pieces in an ovenproof casserole dish. Add salt & pepper.
- Mix the bouillon, wine, and Splenda. Pour over vegetables in the casserole dish and mix well.
- Bake for one hour or until the cabbage is tender.

Makes 8 servings.

TIP: This dish can be reheated in the oven or microwave the following day if there are leftovers.

Nutrition Information per Serving

Calories	68.88
Protein	2.75 g
Carbs	9.84 g
Fat	2.39 g
Fiber	2.95 g
Net carb	6.89 g

Roasted Vegetables

2 medium carrots
1 small turnip
1 medium zucchini
1 medium green pepper
½ cup butternut squash cut
  into bite-sized pieces

1 medium sweet onion
4 tablespoons olive oil
1 tablespoon chopped fresh
  parsley
freshly ground salt & pepper
  to taste

- Preheat oven to 400°.
- Wash and peel carrots. Cut in half lengthwise, then into 1½" pieces.
- Wash and peel turnip and cut into 1½" pieces.
- Peel the onion and cut into 8ths.
- Wash the zucchini and cut in half lengthwise and then into 2" pieces.
- Wash the green pepper, remove seeds, and cut into chunks about 2" in size.
- Combine vegetables in a large bowl with the olive oil and the fresh parsley and toss to coat. Sprinkle with freshly ground pepper & salt.
- Spray a large baking pan with a nonstick product and spoon the vegetables into pan.
- Roast vegetables for 40–50 minutes or until cooked to desired softness, stirring regularly to brown evenly on all sides.

Makes 4 servings.

VARIATION: You may use other vegetables, but keep in mind the carb count will vary. I like to use green beans or asparagus. These vegetables do not take as long to cook as the root vegetables, so I add them only for the last 20 minutes or so.

Nutrition Information per Serving	
Calories	182.80
Protein	1.83 g
Carbs	14.36 g
Fat	14.32 g
Fiber	3.21 g
Net carb	11.05 g

Spaghetti Squash
with Curried Zucchini

1 spaghetti squash
(approximately 3 pounds)
1 cup grated zucchini
2 tablespoons butter
1 tablespoon curry powder

2 tablespoons sour cream
4 tablespoons heavy cream
2 tablespoons chopped fresh
parsley

• Cut the spaghetti squash in half and scoop out seeds with a large spoon. Place the squash cut side down in a large saucepan and add a couple of inches of water. Bring water to a boil, lower the heat, cover pot, and simmer for 20 minutes.
• While the squash is cooking, prepare the zucchini. Grate zucchini with the skin still on and set aside.
• Melt butter over medium heat in a frying pan. Add the curry powder, 2 tablespoons of water, and the grated zucchini. Sauté over medium heat until cooked, about 10 minutes.
• Put the zucchini mixture, sour cream, and heavy cream in a blender and process until smooth. Add the chopped fresh parsley and blend just a bit. Put back in the saucepan to keep warm while you get the spaghetti squash ready.
• Carefully remove the spaghetti squash from the saucepan and place onto a cutting board. Use an oven mitt to hold the squash while you use a fork to scoop out the meat of the squash. It will form spaghetti-like strings. I like to twirl my fork to make attractive little mounds of the squash on the plates.
• Top the squash with the curried zucchini and serve.

Makes 4–6 servings depending on the size of your squash.

Thanks to my friend Jane Gilmore of Toronto, Ontario, who inspired this recipe.

Nutrition Information per Serving	
Calories	151.12
Protein	1.42 g
Carbs	8.73 g
Fat	13.22 g
Fiber	2.30 g
Net carb	6.43 g

Spicy Oven-Baked Zucchini

1 medium zucchini (10–12″ long)
1½ tablespoons olive oil
1 teaspoon Mrs. Dash Extra Spicy

- Preheat oven to 350°.
- Clean and pat dry zucchini. Cut in half lengthwise and then cut into ½″ pieces.
- Place zucchini pieces in a deep bowl and pour olive oil into bowl. Stir to coat with the oil. Add the Mrs. Dash Extra Spicy and stir well to coat the zucchini. Place zucchini on a cookie sheet sprayed with a nonstick agent.
- Bake for 12–15 minutes or until zucchini is soft when a fork is inserted. The zucchini will be brown on the underside.

Makes 2 servings.

Thanks to my daughter-in-law, Sian Haakonson, who inspired this vegetable dish.

Nutrition Information per Serving

Calories	120.22
Protein	1.44 g
Carbs	3.94 g
Fat	10.94 g
Fiber	1.68 g
Net carb	2.26 g

Sweet Tomatoes & Cabbage

2 medium ripe tomatoes

2 packets Splenda

½ cup thinly sliced sweet onion

1 cup sliced cabbage

2 tablespoons extra virgin olive oil

½ teaspoon ground black pepper

¼ teaspoon salt

• Roughly chop tomatoes into ½″ pieces. Sprinkle tomatoes with Splenda and mix in a bowl. Set aside.

• Heat olive oil over medium heat. Sauté the cabbage and onion for 5 minutes, until just soft.

• Add the tomatoes salt & pepper. Continue to cook for an additional 5 minutes. Turn down heat to low, cover the pot, and simmer for a few minutes. *Makes 4 servings.*

Nutrition Information per Serving

Calories	95.48
Protein	1.25 g
Carbs	7.88 g
Fat	7.36 g
Fiber	1.41 g
Net carb	6.47 g

Vegetables in Balsamic Vinegar

8 large mushrooms, stems removed

8 slices (½") eggplant

1 red onion, cut into quarters

8 asparagus spears

½ cup olive oil

4 tablespoons balsamic vinegar

1 teaspoon dry mustard

2 teaspoons chopped fresh thyme

- Preheat oven to 350°.
- Combine olive oil, vinegar, mustard, and thyme. Place vegetables in a shallow bowl and pour marinade over them, turning to coat.
- Place vegetables in a roasting pan that has been sprayed with a nonstick agent. Brush any marinade that remains in the shallow bowl over the vegetables.
- Bake for 35–40 minutes or until all vegetables are cooked, turning once after 20 minutes or so.

Makes 4 servings.

Nutrition Information per Serving

Calories	301.93
Protein	3.45 g
Carbs	11.67 g
Fat	28.60 g
Fiber	3.75 g
Net carb	7.92 g

Vegetable Medley

1 cup yellow zucchini pieces
1 cup green zucchini pieces
1 medium red onion, sliced
½ red pepper, thinly sliced
1 cup green beans or asparagus spears
1 tablespoon olive oil
salt & freshly ground pepper, to taste

• Clean and trim all vegetables.
• Heat olive oil over medium heat in a heavy frying pan. Add vegetables with salt & pepper and sauté for 4–6 minutes, until tender.
Makes 4 servings.

Nutrition Information per Serving	
Calories	66.86
Protein	1.68 g
Carbs	8.27 g
Fat	3.79 g
Fiber	2.81 g
Net carb	5.46 g

Zucchini Ribbons

2 medium zucchini
½ medium onion, thinly sliced
1 cup cherry or grape tomatoes
1½ tablespoons olive oil
¼ teaspoon dried thyme leaves
½ teaspoon freshly ground pepper

- Using a vegetable peeler, slice zucchini into long ribbons.
- Heat olive oil in a large frying pan on medium heat. Add onions and zucchini, sprinkle with thyme and pepper, and sauté for 5 minutes, stirring constantly. Add the tomatoes and continue to cook for another 2–3 minutes. *Makes 4 servings.*

Thanks to my friend Dixie Trenholm of Carp, Ontario, who inspired this dish.

Nutrition Information per Serving

Calories	74.49
Protein	1.67 g
Carbs	6.21 g
Fat	5.54 g
Fiber	1.83 g
Net carb	4.38 g

Zucchini with Tomatoes

3 medium zucchini (about 1½ pounds)
2 tablespoons olive oil
1 medium red onion, quartered and thinly sliced
½ cup white wine
2 medium tomatoes, coarsely chopped
1 tablespoon each chopped fresh parsley & thyme
1 clove garlic, minced
½ teaspoon freshly ground pepper
1 packet Splenda

• In a small bowl, combine tomatoes, garlic, parsley, thyme, and pepper. Sprinkle with Splenda and toss to coat. Let stand for 15 minutes.
• Cut zucchini in half lengthwise and then into ½" slices.
• In a large frying pan, heat oil over medium-high heat. Cook zucchini and onion in oil for 2–3 minutes, until just beginning to brown. Add the wine, reduce heat, and simmer for 5 minutes, until the zucchini is soft and the wine is reduced by half.
• Add the tomato mixture to the zucchini and cook until heated through, about 2 minutes.
Makes 4 servings.

Nutrition Information per Serving	
Calories	109.86
Protein	2.79 g
Carbs	9.41 g
Fat	7.42 g
Fiber	2.90 g
Net carb	6.51 g

POULTRY

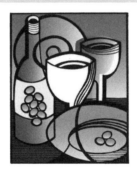

Baked Balsamic Chicken

4 boneless, skinless chicken breasts
3 tablespoons balsamic vinegar
2 tablespoons olive oil
2 cloves garlic, finely minced
freshly ground pepper, to taste

- Preheat over to 375°.
- Combine vinegar, oil, garlic, and pepper to make marinade. Pour over chicken breasts in a shallow bowl, toss to coat, and marinate for 30–45 minutes.
- Spray baking pan with a nonstick agent. Bake the chicken for 40–45 minutes, until done through.

Makes 4 servings.

Nutrition Information per Serving	
Calories	209.19
Protein	29.20 g
Carbs	1.25 g
Fat	8.51 g
Fiber	0.13 g
Net carb	1.12 g

Chicken Breasts with Peppers & Mushrooms

4 boneless, skinless chicken breasts
1 green pepper, thinly sliced
1 medium sweet onion, thinly sliced
2 cups fresh mushrooms, sliced
1 tablespoon olive oil
½ cup chicken bouillon
1 tablespoon butter
¼ cup white wine or sherry
¼ cup heavy cream
1 tablespoon each chopped fresh rosemary & thyme
1 teaspoon freshly ground pepper

- In a large nonstick frying pan, heat oil over medium-high heat and brown chicken on both sides. Remove chicken and place in a warm oven (about 250°).
- Reduce heat to medium and add butter and herbs to the pan. Sauté onions, peppers, and mushrooms until soft, approximately 3–4 minutes.
- Add the chicken stock and wine and bring to a boil. Replace chicken in the pan and cover and simmer for approximately 5 minutes.
- Remove chicken and vegetables and set aside in a warm oven. Add heavy cream and freshly ground pepper. Bring to a vigorous boil, reduce heat, and simmer for 3–4 minutes, until liquid is reduced and sauce has thickened. You may need to add 1 teaspoon of cornstarch, dissolved in a small amount of water, to thicken the sauce.
- Return chicken and vegetables to the pan and continue simmering for 2–3 minutes, turning chicken to coat.
- Top the chicken breasts with vegetables and cream sauce and serve.

Makes 4 servings.

Nutrition Information per Serving	
Calories	294.38
Protein	30.98 g
Carbs	5.77 g
Fat	13.72 g
Fiber	1.29 g
Net carb	4.48 g

Chicken Breasts
with Vegetable Medley

4 boneless, skinless chicken
  breasts
2 tablespoons olive oil
1 medium onion, halved and
  thinly sliced
1 sweet red pepper, halved and
  sliced
2 garlic cloves, minced
1 cup chicken bouillon

12–16 asparagus spears cut into
  2″ pieces
2 medium zucchini, halved and
  cut into ½″ pieces
1 teaspoon freshly ground pepper
½ teaspoon salt
½ teaspoon dried thyme, divided
1 tablespoon chopped fresh
  parsley, to garnish

- Preheat oven to 375°.
- Season chicken breasts with salt, pepper, and half the thyme.
- Heat oil in a large frying pan over medium-high heat. Add chicken and brown well on both sides, about 3 minutes a side. Remove chicken from pan and place in a casserole dish.
- Sauté garlic, onion, pepper, and zucchini for 2–3 minutes, until just soft. Add the asparagus spears and continue cooking for 1 minute. Additional olive oil may be added if necessary.
- Add the chicken bouillon and bring to a boil. Season with additional pepper if desired and the remaining thyme.
- Pour mixture over chicken in the casserole dish and bake, covered, for 20–25 minutes.
- Serve, distributing the vegetables evenly, and garnish with the chopped parsley.

Makes 4 servings.

Nutrition Information per Serving	
Calories	247.69
Protein	31.66 g
Carbs	8.36 g
Fat	9.04 g
Fiber	2.55 g
Net carb	5.81 g

Chicken Cacciatore

3–4 pounds cut-up chicken

½ teaspoon salt

½ teaspoon black pepper

1–2 tablespoons olive oil

1 medium red onion, minced

2 garlic cloves, minced

4 cups sliced fresh mushrooms

1 large can (28 ounces) diced tomatoes

3–4 tablespoons tomato paste

1 cup chicken broth

1 teaspoon dried oregano (not ground but leaves)

1 teaspoon dried basil

½ teaspoon cayenne pepper

2 bay leaves

¼ cup red wine

8–10 cups cooked spinach

• Cut the chicken into reasonable-sized portions. Trim all visible fat and skin. You may use all thighs or all breasts if you wish or buy a whole cut-up chicken.

• Sprinkle chicken with salt and black pepper and brown in hot olive oil over medium heat in a large nonstick skillet or ovenproof stew pot. This may have to be done in batches. Remove chicken from pot and set aside.

• Add onion, garlic, mushrooms, and green pepper to the pot and sauté for approximately 5 minutes or until soft. You may need to add the second table-spoon of olive oil at this point.

continued

- Stir in the chicken broth, being sure to loosen any brown spots at the bottom of the pot. Add the diced tomatoes and tomato paste, stirring to blend. Add the spices and bay leaves.
- Return chicken to the pot. The tomato sauce should almost completely cover the chicken. Place in a 350° oven for 1 hour or until the chicken is tender.
- Remove the pot from the oven and add red wine. If the sauce is a little thin, you may add an additional tablespoon of tomato paste at this point. Return to oven for an additional 30–40 minutes.
- Serve over a bed of steamed spinach.

This dish serves 8.

NOTE: This is a somewhat spicy version of the traditional Italian dish. It freezes well or keeps in the fridge overnight for lunch or dinner the following day.

Nutrition Information per Serving

Calories	555.10
Protein	47.19 g
Carbs	16.51 g
Fat	34.36 g
Fiber	7.69 g
Net carb	8.82 g

Chicken & Mushroom Casserole

4 cups cooked chicken, cut into bite-sized pieces

2 cups sliced fresh mushrooms

2 teaspoons butter

1 cup toasted blanched almonds, whole or slivered

2½ cups White Sauce (see recipe)

½ cup shredded cheese, either cheddar, Swiss, or mozzarella

- Preheat oven to 325°.
- Sauté the mushrooms in butter over medium heat until soft, approximately 4–5 minutes. Set aside.
- Put the cut-up chicken, toasted almonds, and mushrooms in a large bowl.
- Cool the White Sauce slightly and pour over the chicken mixture and blend well. Pour into a 2-quart casserole dish and bake covered for 35 minutes.
- Remove cover and sprinkle with the shredded cheese and continue baking for 15 minutes or until cheese is melted and browned. Serve immediately.

Makes 6 servings.

TIP: This casserole may be made 3–4 hours in advance up to the stage where the white sauce is mixed with the chicken mixture and poured into the casserole dish. You may then put it in the fridge until 1 hour before serving. It may take a few minutes longer in the oven because it was chilled.

TIP: I buy a 3-pound rotisserie chicken at the supermarket to provide the cooked chicken. It allows a nice mix of light and dark meat and saves time.

NOTE: This is an old family favorite that my mother used to make. She used to top it with buttered bread crumbs, which doesn't work for low-carb cooking, but the cheese topping is a nice variation.

Nutrition Information per Serving

Calories	515.02
Protein	30.71 g
Carbs	11.32 g
Fat	39.63 g
Fiber	2.81 g
Net carb	8.51 g

Chicken Roulade

4 boneless, skinless chicken breasts
8 large spinach leaves
1 small zucchini
1 small carrot
4 tablespoons butter, divided
1 teaspoon chopped fresh rosemary
1 teaspoon chopped fresh thyme
1 teaspoon freshly ground pepper
½ teaspoon salt
½ cup sherry
kitchen string

• Pound the chicken breasts flat between two sheets of waxed paper. (I remove the little fillet on the side, which makes it easier to flatten the breast. I use my rolling pin to pound flat.) Set aside.
• Finely shred the zucchini and carrot and set aside.
• Wash the spinach leaves and cook in a saucepan over high heat for 1 minute, using only the water that clings to the leaves. Remove from the pan and place on a paper towel to drain.
• Put 2 tablespoons of the butter in a large frying pan and sauté the zucchini and carrot with salt, pepper, and fresh herbs over medium heat for 3–4 minutes, until soft.
• Lay the flattened chicken breasts on a clean sheet of waxed paper, with the smooth side down. Place two of the cooked spinach leaves on each breast, to cover the exposed side. Take a spoonful of the zucchini and carrot mixture and smooth a thin layer over the spinach leaves.

continued

- Slowly and carefully roll up each breast and tie together at each end with the kitchen string. At this point, the chicken may be covered with clear wrap and put into the fridge until 20 minutes before serving, if desired. This can be done 2–3 hours ahead of time.
- Put 2 tablespoons of butter into a large frying pan over medium-high heat and brown rolled chicken on all sides (4–6 minutes). Add the sherry and bring to a boil. Reduce heat, cover the pan, and simmer chicken for 15 minutes, turning once.
- Remove chicken from frying pan to a cutting board. Remove the string and cut each breast into 3 slices.
- Serve the chicken in overlapping slices on each plate. This is extremely pleasing to the eye, with the chicken, green spinach, and orange filling in the center.

Makes 4 servings.

NOTE: Although this is a little fussy, it is not difficult, and it is very attractive and tasty. I serve it on special occasions because it looks so appealing.

Thanks to my friend Caroline Thoma, who was a willing taste tester and who suggested the name for this dish.

Nutrition Information per Serving	
Calories	285.52
Protein	29.93 g
Carbs	2.81 g
Fat	13.13 g
Fiber	1.03 g
Net carb	1.78 g

Chicken Stew

·····································

2–3 pound whole chicken, cut up

2 tablespoons olive oil

2 sprigs each fresh thyme, rosemary, & oregano

3 cups chicken bouillon

12–16 pearl onions

2 medium carrots

8 celery sticks, leafy tops included

1 small turnip

2 teaspoons dried thyme

1 tablespoon flour

salt & freshly ground pepper, to taste

- Preheat oven to 350°.
- In a deep 4-quart casserole dish, heat oil over medium heat. Salt & pepper chicken pieces and sprinkle with dried thyme. Brown chicken pieces in hot oil on all sides. Remove from casserole dish and set aside.
- Sauté pearl onions for 2–3 minutes. Put chicken back in casserole dish and add the chicken bouillon and the leafy tops only of the celery. Bring to a boil on the stovetop and then place in the oven for 2 hours.
- One hour before serving, remove casserole dish from oven and add carrot and turnip cut into bite-sized pieces. Remove leafy celery tops and add celery sticks cut into 2″ pieces.
- Add additional chicken bouillon if the stew seems dry or the liquid does not cover all vegetables at this point. Mix the tablespoon of flour with 3 tablespoons of water to dissolve and add to the stew, stirring well to distribute. (This will thicken the sauce.)

continued

- Replace in the oven for final hour of cooking.
- Serve chicken pieces with vegetables and sauce on each plate.

Makes 6–8 servings.

VARIATION: You can add small whole mushrooms to the stew during the last hour of baking.

Nutrition Information per Serving	
Calories	348.12
Protein	26.15 g
Carbs	4.43 g
Fat	24.28 g
Fiber	1.15 g
Net carb	3.28 g

Chicken Tenders

4 boneless, skinless chicken breasts, cut into ½″ strips
2 tablespoons olive oil
¼ cup fine bread crumbs
1 tablespoon flour
¼ teaspoon cayenne
1 teaspoon lemon pepper
¼ teaspoon paprika
1 teaspoon thyme
½ teaspoon salt
Mustard Dipping Sauce (see recipe)

• Preheat oven to 375°.
• Combine the bread crumbs and spices in a small bowl and mix well.
• Put cut chicken pieces into a large bowl. Drizzle with the olive oil and stir to coat well. Sprinkle the spice mixture over the chicken and mix well to coat thoroughly.
• Place chicken on a cookie sheet that has been sprayed with a nonstick agent. Sprinkle any remaining spices on the chicken.
• Bake for 18–20 minutes, turning once. The chicken should be nicely browned.
• Serve with Mustard Dipping Sauce.
Makes 6 servings.

Nutrition Information per Serving	
Calories	242.82
Protein	30.17 g
Carbs	7.09 g
Fat	9.01 g
Fiber	0.64 g
Net carb	6.45 g

Chicken Wrap

4 cabbage leaves
1 cup cooked chicken pieces
  (cubed or thinly sliced)
½ red onion, thinly sliced
½ red pepper, thinly sliced
½ green pepper, thinly sliced
1 tablespoon olive oil

1 tomato, seeded and finely
  minced
½ teaspoon salt
½ teaspoon freshly ground
  pepper
½ cup shredded cheddar cheese

• Rinse the cabbage leaves well and cut out the hard core. Place with ½" water in a microwave dish and set aside.
• Mince the tomato, add the salt & pepper, and place in a small serving dish.
• Grate the cheese and place in small serving dish.
• Place the chicken pieces in another small dish.
• Heat the olive oil and sauté the onion and peppers for approximately 7–10 minutes, until soft. Just before the vegetables are done, place the cabbage leaves in the microwave and cook for 3–4 minutes on high. Put the vegetables in a small serving dish and bring the cabbage leaves and each of the serving dishes to the table.
• To serve, take a single cabbage leaf, line it with chicken, onion, and peppers, add tomato, and sprinkle with grated cheese.
Roll up the leaf, tucking in any stray edges.
Makes 2 servings of two wraps each.

VARIATION: You may substitute cooked beef for the chicken as a variation. You may use lettuce leaves as the wrap and take it with you to the golf course or the office.

Nutrition Information per Serving	
Calories	258.05
Protein	28.25 g
Carbs	12.79 g
Fat	113.23 g
Fiber	3.67 g
Net carb	9.12 g

Chicken with Citrus Cranberry Sauce

4 boneless, skinless chicken breasts

2 tablespoons olive oil

1 tablespoon chopped fresh thyme

½ tablespoon chopped fresh parsley

salt & freshly ground pepper, to taste

Citrus Cranberry Sauce

⅓ cup low-carb Cranberry Sauce (see recipe)

⅓ cup chicken bouillon

¼ cup fresh lemon juice

1½ tablespoons Dijon mustard

2 tablespoons heavy cream

1 tablespoon chopped fresh parsley

• Sprinkle chicken with thyme, parsley, and salt & freshly ground pepper.
• Heat the oil in a heavy skillet over medium heat. Add chicken and brown well on both sides, approximately 3–4 minutes a side. Remove to an ovenproof pan and place in a warm oven (250°).
• Add the Citrus Cranberry Sauce ingredients to the skillet, including the low-carb Cranberry Sauce, stirring constantly to blend well, and bring to a boil. Reduce heat to medium and simmer for about 5–6 minutes, until sauce thickens slightly. Return chicken to skillet, turning to coat, and simmer for an additional 5 minutes.
• Transfer the chicken to plates and spoon the Citrus Cranberry Sauce over the chicken.
Makes 4 servings.

Nutrition Information per Serving	
Calories	244.43
Protein	30.56 g
Carbs	4.79 g
Fat	12.48 g
Fiber	0.49 g
Net carb	4.30 g

Chicken with Creamy Mushroom Sauce

4 boneless, skinless chicken breasts

2 tablespoons butter

2 cups fresh mushrooms, cleaned & thinly sliced

1 cup heavy cream

½ teaspoon dried basil

½ teaspoon dried thyme

freshly ground pepper, to taste

¼ teaspoon Fine Herbs

½ teaspoon cornstarch

1 additional teaspoon Fine Herbs

- Trim any fat from chicken breasts. Place cleaned chicken breasts between waxed paper and pound with rolling pin until slightly flattened.
- Make a spice mixture using the basil, thyme, pepper, and Fine Herbs. Sprinkle both sides of the chicken with the herb mixture.
- Melt 1 tablespoon of the butter in a medium-hot frying pan. Add the chicken and brown on both sides, approximately 3–4 minutes a side, until the juices run clear. Remove the chicken to a baking dish and place in a warm oven (250°).
- Add remaining tablespoon of butter to frying pan. Sauté mushrooms until tender, approximately 3–4 minutes.
- Reduce heat to medium and add the cream to the mushrooms and stir vigorously, loosening any brown spots at the bottom of the pan.

continued

• Add salt & ground pepper, to taste, with the additional teaspoon of Fine Herbs. Reduce heat and simmer for 2–3 minutes. Combine ¼ teaspoon cornstarch with a small amount of water and add to the sauce to thicken, stirring constantly.

• Remove chicken from oven and place in the frying pan for a minute or two, turning to coat with cream sauce.

• Spoon the creamy mushroom sauce over each breast and serve.

Makes 4 servings.

TIP: This rich and delicious dish is best served with a green salad and fresh asparagus or some other green vegetable. If you want to lower the fat content of the sauce, you may use 1/2 cup of light cream with 1/2 cup of heavy cream instead of the full cup of heavy cream.

Nutrition Information per Serving

Calories	410.33
Protein	31.42 g
Carbs	4.16 g
Fat	29.53 g
Fiber	0.52 g
Net carb	3.64 g

Chicken with Herbs & Balsamic Vinegar

4 boneless, skinless chicken breasts

2 tablespoons butter

salt & freshly ground pepper, to taste

1 green onion, finely chopped

1 teaspoon each chopped fresh rosemary, thyme, parsley, chives,
    & oregano

2 tablespoons olive oil

2 tablespoons balsamic vinegar

- Put olive oil in a small bowl and add fresh herbs. Set aside.
- Pound chicken breasts flat between two sheets of waxed paper. Salt & pepper breasts.
- Heat butter in a heavy frying pan over medium heat. Add chicken and sauté to brown on each side, approximately 4 minutes per side. Remove chicken from pan and place in a warm oven (250°).
- Reduce heat and put green onion in the frying pan. Sauté 2–3 minutes. Add the herb mixture and vinegar to the pan and continue cooking the herbs and onion to reduce the liquid by half.
- Put chicken breasts on plates and top with herbs in vinegar.

Makes 4 servings.

Nutrition Information per Serving	
Calories	342.94
Protein	54.60 g
Carbs	0.57 g
Fat	11.91 g
Fiber	0.07 g
Net carb	0.50 g

Chicken with Lemon & Mint

4 boneless, skinless chicken breasts
1 teaspoon lemon zest
¼ cup lemon juice
1 tablespoon olive oil
2 cloves garlic, minced
2 tablespoons chopped fresh mint
1 tablespoon chopped fresh thyme
½ teaspoon ground cumin

• Remove any fat from chicken breasts and place in a shallow baking dish.
• Blend lemon juice, zest, olive oil, and herbs together in a small bowl. Pour over chicken and turn chicken to coat. Marinate in fridge for 1 hour.
• Heat grill to medium and place chicken on grill. Cook for 5–6 minutes per side, depending on thickness, until juices run clear.
Makes 4 servings.

Nutrition Information per Serving

Calories	246.88
Protein	29.35 g
Carbs	2.37 g
Fat	12.13 g
Fiber	0.41 g
Net carb	1.96 g

Coq au Vin

3-pound roasting chicken, cut up

2 tablespoons butter

6 slices bacon, diced

8–10 whole small mushrooms

12–16 pearl onions or regular small onions, peeled

½ cup sliced green onion

1 clove garlic, finely minced

3 celery tops with leaves

1½ tablespoons flour

1 teaspoon salt

1 teaspoon freshly ground pepper

1 teaspoon dried thyme

2 cups chicken bouillon

1 cup white wine

- Clean and pat dry chicken pieces.
- In a Dutch oven, over medium heat, sauté bacon until crisp and remove from pan. Add butter to bacon drippings in pan and brown chicken well on all sides. Remove chicken from pan and set aside.
- Pour off all but 2 tablespoons of the fat and add mushrooms and onions and cook until tender and browned. Remove from pan. Add garlic and sauté for 2–3 minutes.
- Remove pan from heat and add flour, salt, pepper, and thyme. Return pan to heat and cook stirring constantly until flour is browned, about 3 minutes.
- Gradually add the chicken bouillon and wine, stirring constantly. Bring mixture to a boil.

continued

- Remove from heat and add bacon, mushrooms & onions, chicken, and celery stalks. Let cool and place in the fridge for 2–3 hours.
- Preheat oven to 400°.
- Bake chicken in covered Dutch oven for approximately 1½–2 hours, until chicken is tender but not falling apart. Remove celery sticks before serving. *Makes 8 servings.*

NOTE: The pearl onions are a bit fussy but well worth the effort in terms of taste and presentation. Use either the pearl onions or the regular small onions but not both.

Nutrition Information per Serving

Calories	550.29
Protein	41.21 g
Carbs	7.59 g
Fat	36.22 g
Fiber	1.62 g
Net carb	5.97 g

Crispy Oven-Baked Chicken

4 chicken breasts (bone in and skin on)
3 tablespoons Crisco cooking oil
1 teaspoon Lawry's Seasoned Salt
1 teaspoon freshly ground pepper
1 teaspoon Fine Herbs
½ teaspoon paprika

- Preheat oven to 400°.
- Combine cooking oil and seasonings in a small bowl. Clean and pat dry chicken breasts. Brush both sides of chicken breasts with the oil mixture.
- Place chicken breasts, skin side up, in a baking dish sprayed with a nonstick agent.
- Bake for 45–55 minutes, depending on the thickness of the breasts, until the skin is browned and crispy and the juices run clear when pierced.
Makes 4 servings.

TIP: This recipe can be made with other chicken parts, including legs, thighs, and wings, with an adjustment in the baking time according to the portion sizes.

My cousin Margot Tompkins gets credit for this easy and delicious recipe, which tastes like fried chicken with none of the hassle of deep-frying.

Nutrition Information per Serving	
Calories	246.26
Protein	33.19 g
Carbs	3.90 g
Fat	13.73 g
Fiber	0.18 g
Net carb	3.72 g

Curried Chicken

4 boneless, skinless chicken
   breasts, cut into 1″ pieces
3 tablespoons olive oil
¼ teaspoon mustard seeds
¼ teaspoon cumin seeds
2 teaspoons curry powder

1 medium onion, thinly sliced
2 cloves garlic, minced
1 teaspoon chopped fresh parsley
1 can (14 ounces) coconut milk
½ cup trimmed green beans
½ cup unsalted whole cashews

• Cut the beans into 1″ pieces and cook with water in the microwave for 2 minutes. Remove from water and set aside.
• In a large nonstick frying pan, heat the olive oil over medium heat. Add the cut-up chicken and brown on all sides. This will take 5–7 minutes. Remove chicken to an ovenproof dish and keep in a warm oven (250°).
• Put the garlic, mustard seed, cumin seed, curry powder, and parsley in the frying pan and sauté for 2–3 minutes. Add the sliced onion and continue cooking until the onion is soft, about 3–4 minutes.
• Stir in the coconut milk and bring to a boil. Reduce heat and add the chicken, cashews, and green beans to the pan. Cook until sauce thickens and chicken and beans are warmed through. You may need to add a teaspoon of cornstarch, dissolved in a small amount of water, to thicken the sauce.
• Serve over a bed of cooked thinly sliced green cabbage.

Makes 4 servings.

TIP: This is a fairly light curry. To increase the heat, simply increase the amount of curry powder.

Nutrition Information per Serving	
Calories	368.95
Protein	32.84 g
Carbs	11.30 g
Fat	21.00 g
Fiber	2.38 g
Net carb	8.92 g

Grilled Herb Chicken

4 boneless, skinless chicken breasts

3 tablespoons fresh lemon juice

3 tablespoons olive oil

2 tablespoons chopped fresh oregano

1 tablespoon chopped fresh parsley

1 tablespoon chopped fresh chives

1 teaspoon freshly ground pepper

½ teaspoon salt

½ teaspoon paprika

• Whisk together olive oil, lemon juice, oregano, parsley, chives, paprika, and salt & pepper. Pour over chicken in a shallow bowl and turn to coat. Let stand for 30–45 minutes in the fridge.

• Heat grill to medium-high heat. Place chicken on grill and close lid. Cook for 4–5 minutes on each side until juices run clear and chicken is cooked through. The cooking time will vary with the size and thickness of the chicken breasts. *Makes 4 servings.*

Nutrition Information per Serving	
Calories	240.19
Protein	29.31 g
Carbs	2.35 g
Fat	12.17 g
Fiber	0.30 g
Net carb	2.05 g

Lemon Herb Chicken

4 boneless, skinless chicken breasts
Lemon Herb Marinade (see recipe)

- Cut any fat off chicken breasts and pat dry.
- Pour marinade over chicken in a shallow bowl. Turn to coat and let stand in the fridge for 1 hour.
- Heat grill or BBQ to medium high. Grill chicken breasts for 4–5 minutes a side, until juices run clear.

Makes 4 servings.

Nutrition Information per Serving

Calories	285.41
Protein	28.88 g
Carbs	1.41 g
Fat	18.19 g
Fiber	0.13 g
Net carb	1.28 g

Lemon Thyme Chicken

4 boneless, skinless chicken breasts
Lemon Thyme Marinade (see recipe)

- Pour marinade over chicken in a shallow bowl and turn to coat. Let stand for 15 minutes.
- Heat grill to medium-high heat. Place chicken on grill and close lid. Cook for 4–5 minutes on each side until juices run clear and chicken is cooked through. Cooking time will vary with the size and thickness of the chicken breasts.
Makes 4 servings.

Nutrition Information per Serving

Calories	151.20
Protein	29.44 g
Carbs	2.21 g
Fat	1.81 g
Fiber	0.34 g
Net carb	1.87 g

Orange Chicken

4 boneless, skinless chicken breasts
Orange Marinade (see recipe)

• Pour marinade over chicken breasts in a shallow bowl and turn to coat. Marinate in the fridge for an hour.
• Preheat the grill to medium high. Place marinated breasts on grill and cook for 4–5 minutes a side, until done. You may also use a frying pan, but it will usually take a bit longer to cook the chicken.
Makes 4 servings.

Nutrition Information per Serving	
Calories	213.18
Protein	29.87 g
Carbs	2.19 g
Fat	8.62 g
Fiber	0.05 g
Net carb	2.14 g

Pecan Chicken with Dijon Sauce

4 boneless, skinless chicken
  breasts
2 tablespoons olive oil
¾ cup finely chopped pecans
1 tablespoon chopped fresh
  thyme
2 tablespoons chopped fresh
  parsley
1 teaspoon freshly ground
  pepper

½ teaspoon salt
½ teaspoon cayenne
½ teaspoon dry mustard
1 egg

Dijon Sauce
½ cup sour cream
2 tablespoons grainy Dijon
  mustard
pinch of salt

- In a small bowl, mix sour cream, mustard, and salt to make the sauce. Serve sauce on the side.
- Whisk together, in a shallow bowl, pecans, parsley, thyme, salt, cayenne, and dry mustard. Set aside.
- In a separate bowl, beat egg.
- Pound chicken breast flat with a rolling pin, between sheets of waxed paper, until they are half their normal thickness.
- Dip each chicken breast in the beaten egg and then in the pecan mixture, coating both sides and pressing into the chicken.
- Heat oil over medium-high heat in a heavy nonstick skillet. Cook chicken, turning once, for approximately 10–12 minutes, until no longer pink inside. If nuts start to get too brown, reduce heat and cook for a few minutes longer.
Makes 4 servings.

Nutrition Information per Serving	
Calories	435.03
Protein	32.08 g
Carbs	5.26 g
Fat	31.45 g
Fiber	2.28 g
Net carb	2.98 g

Quick Chicken Stir-Fry

2 boneless, skinless chicken breasts

2 tablespoons olive oil

2 cups cabbage, thinly sliced

½ sweet onion, minced

1 cup sliced mushrooms

½ cup sliced celery

½ cup chopped asparagus spears

½ medium sweet red pepper, chopped

Oriental Stir-Fry Sauce (see recipe)

½ cup commercial BBQ or stir-fry sauce with ½ cup water

• Heat olive oil in a nonstick pan. Cut the chicken into 1″ cubes and add to the pan. Brown chicken on all sides.

• Add the onion and mushroom and continue to sauté until soft. Add the chopped vegetables and continue cooking for 2–3 minutes.

• Mix the water and prepared sauce to blend. Add the sauce to the stir-fry and continue cooking for a couple of minutes. Alternatively, you may make the Oriental Stir-Fry Sauce and add it to the stir-fry. Cover the pan and let simmer for 3 or 4 minutes.

• Steam cabbage until it is just done, approximately 5 minutes. Drain the cabbage if necessary and mound in the middle of the plate.

• Heap the chicken stir-fry over the cabbage.

Makes 2 servings.

VARIATION: Delete the chicken and add extra low-carb vegetables to make a vegetarian stir-fry.

NOTE: The nutrition calculation does *not* include the sauce in this recipe due to the wide variation possible. Be careful about the carb count on the prepared sauce that you use. A good sauce, if you have a few extra minutes, is our Oriental Stir-Fry Sauce as noted in the recipe.

Nutrition Information per Serving	
Calories	355.11
Protein	33.90 g
Carbs	20.10 g
Fat	16.70 g
Fiber	7.05 g
Net carb	13.05 g

Ricotta Stuffed Chicken Breasts

4 chicken breasts with bone in, skin optional

300 grams ricotta cheese

4 small green onions, chopped

2 cloves garlic, finely chopped

¼ cup chopped fresh cilantro (or flat parsley)

4 fresh rosemary sprigs

4 fresh sage leaves

4 slices bacon

- Preheat oven to 350°.
- In a small bowl, combine the cheese, green onion, garlic, and cilantro. Be sure to blend well.
- Using a sharp knife, cut a slice into the thickest portion of the chicken breast to make an opening. Stuff the opening with the cheese filling. Lay a sprig of rosemary on top of the filling, inside the opening.
- Wrap the chicken breast with a slice of bacon. You can secure the bacon with a toothpick, if necessary. Lay a fresh sage leaf on top of the chicken breast and under the bacon.
- Bake for 40–45 minutes or until the internal temperature of the chicken breast (not the stuffing) is 170° Fahrenheit.

Place the chicken breast under a hot broiler for 2–3 minutes, until the bacon strip is brown and crispy.

Makes 4 servings.

Thanks to Kevin Chenger of Calgary, Alberta, for this great chicken dish.

Nutrition Information per Serving

Calories	336.78
Protein	50.16 g
Carbs	3.73 g
Fat	13.28 g
Fiber	0.25 g
Net carb	3.48 g

Roast Chicken with Lemon & Rosemary

1 whole roasting chicken, about 3 pounds
1 tablespoon olive oil
2 wedges fresh lemon
4 sprigs fresh rosemary
4 sprigs fresh oregano
4 sprigs fresh lemon thyme
1 teaspoon dried rosemary
1 teaspoon dried thyme

• Preheat oven to 350°.
• Clean and pat dry chicken.
• Put lemon wedges and 2 sprigs each of the fresh herbs in the chicken cavity.
• Baste the skin with olive oil and sprinkle the dried herbs over the chicken. Tuck remaining fresh herbs around the wings and legs.
• Roast the chicken for 2½ hours (using ¾ hour per pound due to lemon wedges in cavity) or longer depending on size. Remove from oven and remove all fresh herbs and lemon wedges before carving.
Makes 6–8 servings.

Nutrition Information per Serving

Calories	387.91
Protein	61.39 g
Carbs	0.48 g
Fat	13.34 g
Fiber	0.27 g
Net carb	0.21 g

Spicy Chicken Wings

2 pounds chicken wings or drumettes

2 tablespoons olive oil

2 teaspoons Lawry's Seasoned Salt

2 teaspoons citrus & pepper seasoning

1 teaspoon paprika

1 teaspoon cayenne

1 teaspoon ground thyme

- Wash and pat dry chicken wings or drumettes and place in a bowl. Pour olive oil over chicken and toss to coat thoroughly.
- Blend all spices together in a small dish, sprinkle over chicken parts, and toss to coat. Use hands to rub spices into chicken skin.
- Place on a medium grill and grill 6–7 minutes a side. The chicken may also be baked in a hot oven (375°) for approximately 20 minutes, turning after 10 minutes.

Makes 4 servings, as a meal.

TIP: You may want to use Mustard Dipping Sauce (see recipe) to dip the spicy wings. These are best served with a large green salad.

This is one of two recipes inspired by my daughter-in-law Sian Haakonson.

Nutrition Information per Serving	
Calories	467.25
Protein	61.65 g
Carbs	1.70 g
Fat	22.17 g
Fiber	0.43 g
Net carb	1.27 g

Turkey-Beef Burgers

½ pound lean ground turkey

½ pound lean ground beef

4 tablespoons minced red onion

2 cloves garlic, minced

1 egg

1 teaspoon tomato paste

1 teaspoon Worcestershire Sauce

½ teaspoon paprika

½ teaspoon cayenne

¼ teaspoon ground cumin

salt & freshly ground pepper, to taste

- Combine beef and turkey in a large bowl.
- In a separate bowl, combine the egg with tomato paste, Worcestershire Sauce, and spices.
- Add the onion, garlic, and egg mixture to the meat. Blend well.
- Divide into 4 portions and form patties.
- Place on a hot grill and cook 4–5 minutes on each side, for well done, or until desired doneness.
- You may baste with BBQ sauce, if desired.
This will increase the carbohydrates.

Makes 4 servings.

Nutrition Information per Serving	
Calories	279.65
Protein	28.53 g
Carbs	3.58 g
Fat	16.38 g
Fiber	0.52 g
Net carb	3.06 g

Turkey Burgers

1 pound ground turkey
1 tablespoon minced fresh thyme
½ tablespoon minced fresh rosemary
1 tablespoon minced fresh parsley
1 tablespoon minced fresh chives
1 small egg, slightly beaten
¼ cup fine bread crumbs
¼ cup chopped green onion
1 teaspoon freshly ground pepper
½ teaspoon salt

• Combine all the ingredients in a bowl and mix well. Divide into four portions and make patties.
• Preheat grill to medium high. Place burgers on grill and cook 6–7 minutes a side, until done through.
Makes 4 servings.

**Nutrition Information
per Serving**

Calories	221.35
Protein	22.78 g
Carbs	6.46 g
Fat	11.10 g
Fiber	0.55 g
Net carb	5.91 g

Turkey Loaf

1½ pounds ground turkey (½ breast & ½ thigh)
¼ cup fine bread crumbs
1 egg, slightly beaten
⅓ cup red onion, minced
½ cup celery, minced
2 medium mushrooms, minced
½ cup chicken bouillon
1 teaspoon Fine Herbs
salt & freshly ground pepper, to taste

- Preheat oven to 350°.
- Mix all ingredients in a large bowl. Place into loaf pan and press with spoon. Sprinkle top with additional ½ teaspoon Fine Herbs and cover with foil.
- Bake for 55 minutes and remove foil. Bake an additional 5 minutes.
Makes 6 servings.

NOTE: This loaf is somewhat pale in color but very tasty. You may wish to add some low-carb Cranberry Sauce as a garnish. Remember that this will slightly increase the carbohydrates.

Nutrition Information per Serving

Calories	207.57
Protein	22.01 g
Carbs	4.85 g
Fat	10.66 g
Fiber	0.48 g
Net carb	4.37 g

Turkey Stuffing

6 slices low-carb bread
2 cups cabbage cut into 1″ pieces
1 cup shredded carrot
1 cup chopped celery
1 small sweet onion, minced
1 cup chopped walnuts
½ teaspoon ground sage

1 teaspoon poultry seasoning
1 teaspoon Fine Herbs
½ teaspoon dried oregano leaves
½ teaspoon dried thyme leaves
½ teaspoon parsley
½ teaspoon black pepper
¼ teaspoon salt

- Dry the bread overnight or for 15–20 minutes in a low oven. Break the bread into small cubes. You should have approximately 6 cups.
- Prepare the vegetables and add to the bread crumbs. Sprinkle with spices and mix well with hands to distribute the spices.
- Stuff the turkey cavity and bake as per instructions for the bird.
- This will make enough stuffing for a 10–12-pound turkey.

Makes 20 servings of ½ cup each.

TIP: For additional flavor, and to further reduce the carb content, replace some of the cabbage with chopped pork rinds.

NOTE: The carb content will vary with the bread used. For this recipe, I found and used a sugar-free whole wheat bread that had 11 carbs per slice. Since I developed this recipe, there are now many low-carb breads lower in carb content, and using one of these breads will decrease the total carbs for the stuffing. This dressing stays nice and moist thanks to the vegetables.

Nutrition Information per Serving

Calories	56.91
Protein	2.10 g
Carbs	5.08 g
Fat	3.83 g
Fiber	1.03 g
Net carb	4.05 g

White Chicken Chili

....

4 boneless, skinless chicken breasts

4 cups chicken bouillon

1 large sweet onion, roughly chopped

1 large cauliflower

1 garlic clove, minced

2 tablespoons butter

2 celery stalks chopped, with leafy tops separated

2 cups fresh green beans cut into ½″ pieces

1 green pepper, chopped

1 teaspoon ground cumin

1 teaspoon cayenne pepper

2 bay leaves

1 teaspoon salt

1 cup chicken broth, if required

2 teaspoons cornstarch dissolved in 4 teaspoons water

chopped fresh parsley, to garnish

• Place the chicken breasts with the water and chicken bouillon in a large Dutch oven or stew pot. Add the leafy tops of the celery ribs and approximately one-third of the chopped onion. Cook over medium-high heat until the chicken is cooked through, approximately 20 minutes.

• Remove the chicken from the pot and reserve the broth. Discard the leafy tops of the celery ribs. Put the cauliflower, cut into small florets, into the broth and cook until soft. This will take 15–20 minutes.

continued

- While the cauliflower is cooking, cut chicken into bite-sized pieces and set aside.
- Melt the butter in a frying pan over medium heat. Add the remaining onion, celery, garlic, and green pepper. Sauté vegetables for approximately 5 minutes, until soft.
- Using an immersion blender, process the cauliflower in the broth. If you do not have an immersion blender, this may be done in a food processor.
- You now have a slightly thickened white sauce. Put in the chicken pieces, sautéed vegetables, green beans, bay leaves, and spices. Stir to blend well. Do not add the chopped parsley until serving.
- Place in a 350° oven for up to 2 hours, until the sauce is further thickened. The liquid should fully cover the chicken and all the vegetables. You may add a little extra chicken broth, if necessary. You may need to add the cornstarch and water 30 minutes before serving, if the sauce has not thickened enough.
- Serve in big bowls and top with shredded cheese, salsa, or sour cream. Garnish with freshly chopped parsley. This dish goes well with a fresh green salad.

Makes 4 servings.

NOTE: This is a great southern twist on the old red chili. It is hot and spicy. You can reduce the cayenne pepper to half, if you find it too hot. The sauce is not as thick as the red variety, but it has a wonderful flavor all its own.

Nutrition Information per Serving

Calories	259.40
Protein	34.60 g
Carbs	18.70 g
Fat	5.88 g
Fiber	7.26 g
Net carb	11.44 g

FISH

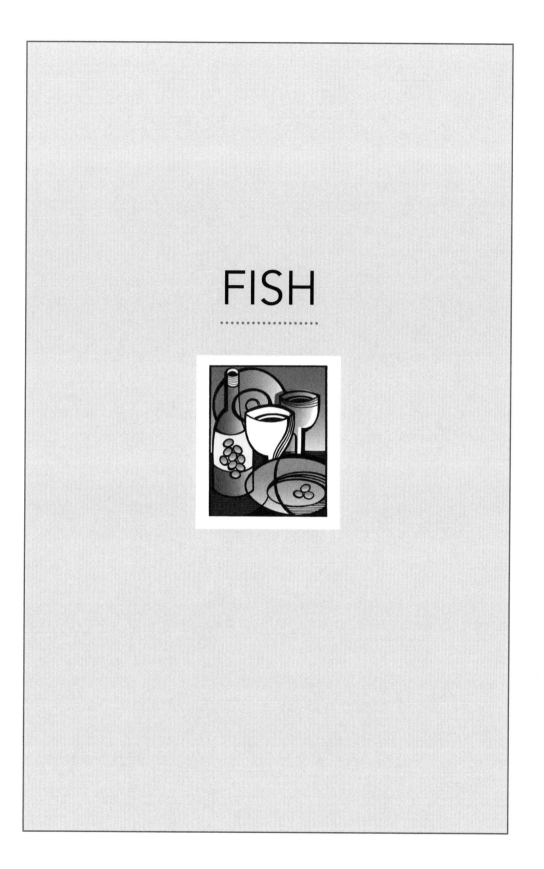

Baked Halibut with Sour Cream

1½ pounds halibut fillet

½ cup chopped green onion

1 cup sour cream

¼ teaspoon ground black pepper

¼ teaspoon dried dill

⅓ cup grated Parmesan cheese

- Preheat oven to 350°.
- Place the halibut in the bottom of a well-buttered baking dish.
- Combine all ingredients except the cheese. Pour this thick, creamy mixture over the halibut.
- Bake for 20–25 minutes, depending on the thickness of your fillet.
- Sprinkle with the finely grated cheese and put under the hot broiler just long enough to brown the cheese.

Makes 6 servings.

Thanks to Valerie Caspersen of Victoria, British Columbia, for this great recipe.

Nutrition Information per Serving

Calories	187.22
Protein	17.86 g
Carbs	3.53 g
Fat	11.11 g
Fiber	0.23 g
Net carb	3.30 g

Baked Sole

4 fillets of sole (4–6 ounces each)

⅓ cup fine bread crumbs

1 teaspoon paprika

½ teaspoon each basil, thyme, oregano, & rosemary

¼ teaspoon cayenne pepper

1 teaspoon freshly ground pepper

⅓ cup whole milk

4 sprigs fresh parsley

4 lemon wedges

- Preheat oven to 350°.
- Mix spices together with bread crumbs in a shallow bowl.
- Dip fillets in whole milk and then coat with seasoned bread crumbs.
- Place fillets in a baking dish sprayed with a nonstick agent. Bake for 10–15 minutes, depending on the thickness of the fillets. To test for doneness, use a fork, and fish will flake easily and be opaque throughout when done.
- Serve with a lemon wedge and a sprig of fresh parsley.

Makes 4 servings.

Nutrition Information per Serving	
Calories	187.92
Protein	30.46 g
Carbs	8.33 g
Fat	2.81 g
Fiber	0.58 g
Net carb	7.75 g

Baked Whole Salmon

1 dressed salmon (2–3 pounds)
4 thin lemon slices
4 thin onion rings
1 tablespoon chopped fresh parsley
½ tablespoon chopped fresh rosemary
¼ cup fresh lemon juice
2 teaspoons butter
salt & freshly ground pepper, to taste

- Preheat oven to 400°. Spray a large baking dish with a nonstick product.
- Salmon should have head removed and interior cavity cleaned. Wash with cold water and pat dry.
- Open the cavity and place layers of lemon slices, onion slices, fresh herbs, and salt & pepper inside. Dot with small amounts of butter.
- Place the salmon in the baking dish and sprinkle with lemon juice. Pour remaining juice in the bottom of the baking dish.
- Bake uncovered for 20–25 minutes, allowing approximately 9–10 minutes per pound, depending on the thickness of the fish. Test with a fork for doneness: the salmon should be evenly pink throughout and flake easily.
- To serve, remove skin and cut sections of fish on either side of the backbone. Serve with a wedge of lemon.

Makes 8–12 servings.

NOTE: This fish presents very well since it is cooked whole. I often bring it to the table on a pretty platter to serve.

Nutrition Information per Serving	
Calories	219.59
Protein	22.66 g
Carbs	1.05 g
Fat	13.08 g
Fiber	0.16 g
Net carb	0.89 g

BBQ'd Salmon with Basil Sauce

1–1½ pounds salmon fillets
4 sprigs fresh dill
8 fresh chives
2 tablespoons white wine
1 teaspoon butter
Basil Sauce (see recipe)

• Grease a large piece of tinfoil with butter. Make sure that you have sufficient tinfoil to tent the salmon fillets. Cut the fillets into four pieces.
• Place the salmon on the tinfoil, skin side down. Place two fresh chives and a sprig of fresh dill on each fillet. Sprinkle with a little freshly ground pepper & salt. Pour the white wine over the fish and fold the tinfoil to make an airtight tent over the salmon.
• Place on a hot BBQ for 12–15 minutes, depending on the thickness of the fillets.
• To serve, pour a couple of tablespoons of sauce over the salmon.
Makes 4 servings.

NOTE: Although there is some saturated fat in the mayonnaise in the sauce, most of the fat in this delicious recipe is from the salmon and is the type of good fat that you want to increase in your diet.

Nutrition Information per Serving

Calories	511.74
Protein	22.99 g
Carbs	3.23 g
Fat	44.35 g
Fiber	0.51 g
Net carb	2.72 g

Broiled Halibut

4 halibut steaks, about 1½" thick (4–6 ounces each)
2 teaspoons butter
2 teaspoons lemon juice
2 teaspoons chopped fresh thyme
1 tablespoon chopped fresh parsley
salt & freshly ground pepper, to taste
4 lemon wedges

- Preheat broiler for 10 minutes.
- Rinse halibut under cold water and pat dry. Place on rack of broiler pan sprayed with a nonstick product.
- Sprinkle with herbs and salt & pepper. Distribute butter evenly in little pats on the halibut and sprinkle with lemon juice.
- Place pan 2" from broiler and broil for 5–6 minutes a side or until fish is no longer opaque and flakes easily with a fork. The broiling time will vary with the thickness of the steaks. Be sure to test for doneness before removing from oven.
- To finish, serve with a fresh lemon wedge and additional chopped fresh parsley sprinkled on the halibut.

Makes 4 servings.

TIP: Although fresh herbs make a difference in taste and presentation, dried herbs may be used, and quantities should be halved in this case.

Nutrition Information per Serving

Calories	146.47
Protein	23.92 g
Carbs	1.20 g
Fat	4.58 g
Fiber	0.27 g
Net carb	0.93 g

Broiled Salmon

4 salmon fillets (about 4–6 ounces each)

2 teaspoons lemon juice

1 teaspoon butter

1 tablespoon each chopped fresh thyme, parsley, & chives

1 teaspoon freshly ground pepper

- Preheat broiler. Spray broiler rack with a nonstick agent.
- Place fillets on broiler pan and sprinkle each fillet with the combined fresh herbs. Put a dot of butter on each fillet and sprinkle with lemon juice.
- Place broiler pan 2″ from broiler and broil for 7–10 minutes, without turning, until cooked through. Test for doneness with a fork: the fish should flake easily and be pink throughout.
- Serve with a lemon wedge.
  Makes 4 servings.

Nutrition Information per Serving	
Calories	253.48
Protein	33.87 g
Carbs	0.68 g
Fat	11.81 g
Fiber	0.16 g
Net carb	0.52 g

Cold Salmon with Dill Sauce

1–1½-pound salmon fillet
½ cup white wine
¼ cup fresh lemon juice
1 tablespoon chopped fresh parsley
1 teaspoon freshly ground pepper
Creamy Dill Sauce (see recipe)

- Preheat oven to 400°. Spray baking pan with a nonstick agent.
- Place salmon in the baking dish (skin down if skin attached). Sprinkle the salmon with the freshly ground pepper and parsley. Add the white wine and lemon juice to the bottom of the pan. Cover the pan with foil and seal the edges.
- Bake for 15–20 minutes, until the fish is cooked through. It will flake easily and be a uniform pink throughout when done. Cooking time will depend on the thickness of the fish.
- Let cool slightly, remove from the pan, and chill in the fridge for at least 2–3 hours. Serve with Creamy Dill Sauce on the side.

Makes 4–6 servings.

Nutrition Information per Serving	
Calories	318.32
Protein	22.82 g
Carbs	2.25 g
Fat	22.51 g
Fiber	0.05 g
Net carb	2.20 g

Crusted Salmon with Rosemary Sour Cream

1½ pounds salmon fillets

2 packets Splenda

2 tablespoons Dijon mustard

1 tablespoon sesame seeds

1 tablespoon yellow mustard seeds

1½ tablespoons chopped fresh rosemary leaves

½ cup sour cream

½ tablespoon chopped fresh parsley

½ tablespoon chopped fresh dill

1 teaspoon ground ginger

1 tablespoon chopped green onion

- Preheat oven to 450°.
- Place salmon fillets, skin side down, on a cookie sheet lined with foil and buttered.
- In a small bowl, mix the mustard and Splenda. Add the mustard seeds, sesame seeds, and chopped fresh rosemary to the mustard mixture. Evenly spread this mixture over the salmon fillets.
- Bake until the salmon is pink throughout, about 10–15 minutes, depending on the thickness of the fillets.
- While the salmon is baking, stir together the sour cream, chopped fresh parsley and dill, and ground ginger.
- Using a spatula, lift the salmon carefully from the cookie sheet. Garnish the salmon with a dollop of the rosemary sour cream and a sprinkle of chopped green onions.

Makes 4 servings.

Nutrition Information per Serving	
Calories	410.36
Protein	35.74 g
Carbs	6.74 g
Fat	26.12 g
Fiber	1.92 g
Net carb	4.82 g

Grilled Halibut

4 halibut steaks, about 1″ thick

3 lemons

2 tablespoons olive oil

2 teaspoons chopped fresh oregano

1 teaspoon chopped fresh chives

1 teaspoon chopped fresh rosemary

1 teaspoon chopped fresh parsley

salt & freshly ground pepper, to taste

• In a small bowl, combine zest of 1 lemon and juice of 2 lemons with olive oil and fresh herbs.

• Rinse halibut under cold water and pat dry. Place in a shallow dish.

• Pour lemon juice and herb marinade over halibut and marinate in fridge for 1 hour.

• Heat grill to medium. Spray a grilling basket with a nonstick product. Place halibut steaks in grilling basket and grill for 3–4 minutes a side or until fish is no longer opaque and flakes easily with a fork. The grilling time will vary with the thickness of the steaks.

• To finish, serve with a fresh lemon wedge and additional chopped fresh parsley sprinkled on the halibut.

• If available, a small mound of cooked sea asparagus (found in the fresh fish department) on each steak makes a dramatic garnish.

Makes 4 servings.

TIP: Although fresh herbs make a difference in taste and appearance, dried herbs may be used, and quantities should be halved in this case.

Nutrition Information per Serving

Calories	265.0
Protein	36.41 g
Carbs	6.49 g
Fat	11.20 g
Fiber	2.64 g
Net carb	3.85 g

Poached Salmon with Citrus Sauce

1–1½ pounds fresh salmon fillet

½ cup fresh orange juice

½ teaspoon ground pepper

¼ teaspoon salt

Citrus Sauce (see recipe)

- Preheat oven to 425°.
- Cut salmon into four equal parts. Place skin side down on a large piece of buttered tinfoil in a baking dish. Sprinkle with salt & pepper.
- Pour fresh orange juice over salmon, fold tinfoil to make a tent, and bake for 8–10 minutes, depending on the thickness of the fillets. You may warm the orange juice in the microwave before pouring over the salmon.
- While salmon is baking, prepare the Citrus Sauce.
- Remove the salmon carefully from the foil tent since it will be full of steam. Let the salmon sit for 2–3 minutes. Place on individual plates and divide the sauce among the servings. Pour the sauce over the salmon.

Makes 4 servings.

NOTE: Do not be distressed by the fat content in this dish. The majority of the fat comes from the salmon, which is full of the "good fats."

Thanks to Linda Porter of Delta, British Columbia, for this wonderful dish.

Nutrition Information per Serving

Calories	408.47
Protein	34.12 g
Carbs	4.22 g
Fat	27.54 g
Fiber	0.02 g
Net carb	4.20 g

Salmon Poached with Vegetables

4 salmon fillets (about 4–6 ounces each) or steaks about 1″ thick
⅔ cup chicken bouillon
1 cup green beans, trimmed (or fresh asparagus)
½ cup julienne carrots
6 sprigs fresh thyme
1 clove garlic, minced
1 cup julienne yellow or green zucchini (or ½ cup each julienne red and green pepper)
⅔ cup white wine
salt & freshly ground pepper, to taste

- Wash all vegetables well and prepare according to ingredients list.
- Preheat oven to 350°.
- In a stove-top and oven-safe casserole dish, combine chicken bouillon, green beans, carrots, thyme, and garlic. Bring to a simmer over medium heat, cover, and cook for 5 minutes. Stir in either zucchini or bell peppers and wine. Simmer for 1 minute and remove from heat.
- Season salmon with salt & pepper. Place salmon over vegetables in pan (if using fillets, place skin side down).
- Cover with lid and bake at 350° for 10–15 minutes, depending on thickness of fish. Fish is done when it flakes easily with a fork and is a uniform pink throughout.
- Discard thyme sprigs. Serve salmon and vegetables on individual plates and garnish with lemon wedge and chopped fresh parsley. Drizzle with cooking liquid.

Makes 4 servings.

Nutrition Information per Serving

Calories	315.93
Protein	40.23 g
Carbs	6.62 g
Fat	10.86 g
Fiber	2.31 g
Net carb	4.31 g

Salmon Poached in White Wine

1½-pound salmon fillet
⅓ cup white wine
⅓ cup fresh lemon juice
4 thin lemon slices
4 rounds sweet onion, thinly sliced
1 tablespoon each chopped fresh rosemary, thyme, & parsley
Lemon Thyme Sauce (see recipe)

- Preheat oven to 400°. Spray baking pan with a nonstick agent.
- You may use a single large piece of fish or 4 fillets — the recipe works either way. Place salmon in the baking dish (skin down if skin attached). Layer the salmon with the fresh herbs, sliced lemon, and sliced onion. Add the white wine and lemon juice to the bottom of the pan. Cover the pan with foil and seal the edges.
- Bake for 15–20 minutes, until the fish is cooked through. The fish will flake easily and be a uniform pink when done.
- Serve with Lemon Thyme Sauce on the side.

Makes 4 servings.

TIP: I usually make more salmon than I need when using this recipe because the salmon is so moist. The next day I make salmon salad with the leftovers.

**Nutrition Information
per Serving**

Calories	285.00
Protein	28.42 g
Carbs	2.71 g
Fat	15.41 g
Fiber	0.36 g
Net carb	2.35 g

Salmon with Balsamic Citrus Sauce

4 salmon fillets (about 4–6 ounces each)
2 teaspoons butter
½ teaspoon salt
½ teaspoon freshly ground pepper
Balsamic Citrus Sauce (see recipe)

- Preheat oven to 450°. Spray a baking pan with a nonstick agent.
- Season the salmon with salt & pepper. Melt 2 teaspoons of butter in a large frying pan over medium-high heat and brown the fillets on both sides. This will take 3 minutes or so for each side.
- Place the salmon in the baking dish. Bake for 7–10 minutes, until the fish is cooked through. The fish will flake easily and be a uniform pink throughout when done.
- While the fish is baking, proceed with the Balsamic Citrus Sauce.
- Remove salmon fillets from oven, place on individual plates, and spoon sauce over the salmon.

Makes 4 servings.

Nutrition Information per Serving

Calories	207.90
Protein	22.68 g
Carbs	1.90 g
Fat	10.12 g
Fiber	0.04 g
Net carb	1.86 g

Shrimp Delight

6 large or jumbo shrimp (raw)
1 tablespoon butter
½ small red onion, thinly sliced
1½ cups sliced fresh mushrooms
1–2 cloves garlic, minced
1 teaspoon freshly ground pepper
1 tablespoon white wine (or sherry)

- Sauté the onion, mushroom, and garlic in butter for about 5 minutes or until nicely soft.
- Add the shrimp and ground pepper and stir until the shells are bright pink.
- Add the white wine (or sherry) just a few minutes before the shrimp are done; then cover and simmer.
- Serve on a lunch plate with a fresh green salad.

Makes 2 servings.

VARIATION: You may substitute olive oil for butter, but the shrimp will not taste quite as rich.

Thanks to Patricia Shaw of North Bay, Ontario, for this great recipe.

Nutrition Information per Serving	
Calories	109.58
Protein	6.78 g
Carbs	6.25 g
Fat	6.41 g
Fiber	1.39 g
Net carb	4.86 g

Sole with Herb Butter

4 sole fillets (4–6 ounces each)
1 tablespoon olive oil
2 tablespoons butter
½ tablespoon each chopped fresh dill, thyme, & mint
1 tablespoon chopped fresh parsley
1 teaspoon freshly ground pepper
½ teaspoon salt
¼ cup whole milk
4 sprigs fresh parsley or dill
4 lemon wedges

• Bring butter to room temperature. Add lemon juice and chopped fresh herbs and mix well with a fork until blended. Form small swirls or patties with the butter, place on waxed paper, and put in the fridge to chill.
• Dip fillets in whole milk. Heat olive oil in a large frying pan over medium-high heat. Sprinkle fillets with freshly ground pepper & salt.
• Place fillets in a frying pan and cook for 3–4 minutes a side until well browned and cooked through. To test for doneness, use a fork: the fish will flake easily and be opaque throughout when done.
• Serve with a pat of herb butter melting on the fillet, a lemon wedge, and a sprig of fresh parsley or dill.
Makes 4 servings.

Nutrition Information per Serving

Calories	229.61
Protein	29.18 g
Carbs	1.63 g
Fat	11.34 g
Fiber	0.42 g
Net carb	1.21 gg

Sole with Herbs & Spices

4 sole fillets (about 1½ pounds)

⅓ cup fine bread crumbs

1 tablespoon flour

¾ teaspoon cayenne

1 teaspoon oregano

1½ teaspoons lemon pepper

½ teaspoon thyme

1 egg, slightly beaten

1 tablespoon olive oil

2 teaspoons freshly chopped parsley

• In a shallow dish, mix together the bread crumbs with all the spices and herbs, except the freshly chopped parsley.

• Dip the fillets in the egg mixture. Coat each fillet with the spice mixture on each side.

• Heat the olive oil in a medium-hot skillet and add the fillets. Sauté for 3–4 minutes on each side, depending on thickness of fillets. Fish is done when browned and it flakes when a fork is inserted.

• Serve with lemon wedges and sprinkle each fillet with the chopped fresh parsley.

Makes 4 servings.

Nutrition Information per Serving	
Calories	235.53
Protein	31.78 g
Carbs	9.30 g
Fat	6.91 g
Fiber	0.56 g
Net carb	8.74 g

Steamed Halibut
with Herbs & Vegetables

4 halibut fillets (4–6 ounces)

3 cups fresh broccoli florets

1 medium carrot, julienned

4 slices thinly sliced onion

2 tablespoons water

2 tablespoons white wine

4 sprigs fresh lemon thyme

4 sprigs fresh parsley

1 teaspoon freshly ground pepper

4 slices lemon

4 wedges lemon

- Preheat oven to 450°.
- Place halibut in a nonstick baking dish. Season halibut with freshly ground pepper and layer with onion slice, lemon slice, and sprigs of fresh herbs. Place broccoli florets and carrots in the dish and add liquid.
- Cover the baking dish with aluminum foil and bake for 10–12 minutes. Test for doneness with a fork. Fish should be white and flaky when done.
- To serve, place fish on plates, removing lemon slice and herb sprigs. Spoon pan juices over halibut. Add vegetables and a wedge of fresh lemon.

Makes 4 servings.

Nutrition Information per Serving	
Calories	181.28
Protein	26.24 g
Carbs	7.38 g
Fat	2.95 g
Fiber	3.03 g
Net carb	4.35 g

MEATS

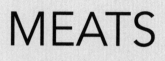

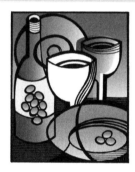

BBQ Spare Ribs

2 racks pork (or beef) back ribs (about 2–3 pounds)
1 small onion, halved
4 cups chicken bouillon
4 celery stalks with leaves on
salt & freshly ground pepper, to taste
BBQ Sauce (see recipe)

- Cut the ribs into sections of 3–4 bones each. Salt & pepper the ribs.
- Fill large stock pot or stew pot with bouillon, leaving just enough room to add the ribs (add water if additional liquid is necessary). Put ribs, onion, and celery tops into pot and bring to a boil. Reduce heat to medium and simmer for 1 hour.
- Remove ribs from pot and cool slightly. Baste the ribs with BBQ Sauce on both sides.
- Preheat BBQ to medium-high heat. Place the ribs on the BBQ and grill until brown and glazed with sauce, about 4–5 minutes a side.

Makes 4 servings.

NOTE: The nutrition information is provided for the ribs only. Add the carb content for whichever BBQ Sauce you use with your ribs.

Nutrition Information per Serving

Calories	405.15
Protein	26.56 g
Carbs	0.00 g
Fat	32.39 g
Fiber	0.00 g
Net carb	0.00 g

Beef Bourguignon

1½–2 pounds lean stewing beef

1 tablespoon butter

1 tablespoon olive oil

4 slices bacon, cut into ½″ pieces

1½ cups beef bouillon

1 tablespoon flour

4 celery stick tops, including leaves

2 teaspoons Fine Herbs

salt & freshly ground pepper, to taste

To Finish

1½ cups small fresh mushrooms, stems removed

½ cup pearl onions, peeled and washed

1 tablespoon butter

¼ cup red wine

- Preheat oven to 325°.
- Cut beef into bite-sized pieces and remove any fat. Season meat with salt & pepper.
- In a large oven- and stove-top-proof casserole dish, heat butter and olive oil over medium heat. Add beef and brown on all sides while stirring constantly. Remove beef from casserole dish and set aside.
- Add bacon to the casserole dish and cook until crisp, approximately 2–3 minutes. Reduce heat and stir in the flour, making sure to loosen any brown bits from the bottom.

continued

- Add beef bouillon, celery tops, Fine Herbs, and beef. Place casserole dish in the oven and simmer at 325° for 2 hours. (Check the casserole and stir after 1 hour. Add additional beef bouillon if the dish is getting dry.)
- To finish, remove casserole dish from oven approximately 35 minutes before serving and remove celery tops and discard.
- Sauté small mushrooms and pearl onions in butter in a frying pan for 2–3 minutes. Add red wine and bring to a boil.
- Add wine with vegetables to the casserole dish and return to the oven to continue simmering for 30 minutes.

Makes 6 servings.

NOTE: The pearl onions are fussy to peel, but they are worth the trouble in terms of taste and presentation.

Nutrition Information per Serving

Calories	342.67
Protein	30.11 g
Carbs	4.06 g
Fat	22.45 g
Fiber	0.67 g
Net carb	3.39 g

Beef Burgers
with Onions & Mushrooms

1 pound lean ground beef

2 teaspoons olive oil

1 medium sweet onion, sliced and separated into rings

1 cup thinly sliced fresh mushrooms

2 teaspoons balsamic vinegar

½ teaspoon salt

1 teaspoon dried thyme

1½ teaspoons paprika

½ teaspoon cayenne

1 teaspoon ground pepper, to taste

- Preheat grill to medium-high heat.
- Combine all spices in a small bowl. Divide meat into four portions and form patties. Coat each side of the patty with spice mixture and press lightly with palms to ensure that spices stick to the patty.
- Place patties on grill and cook over medium-high heat for 4–5 minutes a side, depending on the thickness of the patty. Test for doneness. Burgers should be cooked through.
- While burgers are cooking, heat oil in a large frying pan over medium heat and add onions. Sauté onions until soft, about 3 minutes. Add mushrooms and cook for 5 minutes more, stirring constantly. Add vinegar to the pan and continue cooking for 2 minutes, stirring constantly. Remove from heat and set aside.
- Remove patties from grill and top with equal portions of the onion and mushroom mixture.

Makes 4 servings.

Nutrition Information per Serving	
Calories	296.12
Protein	21.99 g
Carbs	2.76 g
Fat	21.31 g
Fiber	0.84 g
Net carb	1.92 g

Beef Stroganoff

1½ pounds sirloin steak, ½"–1" thick
½ teaspoon salt
½ teaspoon freshly ground pepper
2 tablespoons olive oil
1 large sweet onion, minced
2 cups fresh mushroom slices
2 cups beef broth
1 tablespoon Dijon mustard
1 tablespoon tomato paste
½ cup red wine
1 tablespoon flour
1 teaspoon cornstarch
2 teaspoons water
¾ cup sour cream
6 cups sliced cabbage
1 tablespoon chopped fresh parsley

• Cut steak into thin slices, approximately 1–2" in length. Sprinkle with salt & pepper.
• Heat the olive oil in a large skillet or stew pot. Add the beef strips and brown on all sides. Add the mushrooms and onion and sauté for 5 minutes or until tender.
• Whisk the mustard and tomato paste into the beef broth until dissolved. Add the broth mixture to the beef and vegetables. Cover, reduce heat, and simmer for 45 minutes.

continued

- Cut the cabbage into long strips about a ¼″ thick. The cabbage will take the place of egg noodles. Bring a large pot of water to a boil just 5 minutes before serving. Put the cabbage in the pot and cook for 3–5 minutes. You want the cabbage to be a little firm.
- While the cabbage is cooking, whisk the flour and cornstarch into the wine with water and add to the beef mixture. Add the sour cream and stir to blend. Cook, stirring constantly, until the sauce is thickened.
- Drain the cabbage well. Serve the beef over the hot cabbage and garnish with chopped fresh parsley.

Makes 6 servings.

TIP: This dish, served over a slice of low-carb toast, is delicious the next day for lunch.

Nutrition Information per Serving

Calories	340.28
Protein	24.29 g
Carbs	16.52 g
Fat	18.96 g
Fiber	6.82 g
Net carb	9.70 g

Braised Pork Loin Chops

6 pork chops, center loin
1 small onion, cut in half and thinly sliced
1 tablespoon olive oil
1 tablespoon chopped fresh rosemary
½ teaspoon ground black pepper
¼ teaspoon salt
½ cup sour cream
⅓ cup heavy cream
2 cups sliced mushrooms

• Preheat oven to 350°.
• Trim all visible fat from the chops. Sprinkle half the rosemary and pepper & salt on the chops.
• Brown both sides of the pork chops in the olive oil. This will take 3–4 minutes a side. Remove to a baking pan.
• Sauté the onions and mushrooms until soft in the same pan used to brown the chops. Add the remaining herbs, sour cream, and heavy cream to the vegetable mixture and stir to blend.
• Pour this mixture over the chops and bake for 30–40 minutes, depending on the thickness of the chops, until tender.
Makes 6 servings.

NOTE: This recipe also works well for boneless pork loin and does not need as much time in the oven without the bone.

Nutrition Information per Serving

Calories	263.33
Protein	23.63 g
Carbs	2.40 g
Fat	17.51 g
Fiber	0.35 g
Net carb	2.06 g

Cabbage Rolls

1 small head cabbage
1¼ pound lean ground beef
1 cup finely shredded zucchini
1 celery stick, minced
½ cup finely chopped onions
1 egg
2 tablespoons chopped fresh
   parsley
½ teaspoon salt
1 teaspoon freshly ground pepper

Topping
1 medium onion, minced
½ cup chopped celery
½ cup sliced mushrooms
1 garlic clove, minced
2 tablespoons light olive oil
½ cup water
1 can condensed tomato soup
1 tablespoon chopped fresh
   parsley

- Preheat oven to 350°.
- Remove the core from the cabbage and separate the leaves. Microwave the leaves in ½ cup of water for 5 minutes on high and set aside.
- Combine the beef, minced celery, onion, and zucchini in a large mixing bowl. Beat the egg slightly and add it to the beef, along with the chopped parsley and salt & pepper. Mix thoroughly.
- Place approximately ¼ of a cup of the beef mixture in the middle of each cabbage leaf. Roll up, tucking in any edges to make a tight package, and place in a baking dish sprayed with a nonstick agent. Repeat until all beef is used.
- Sauté garlic, remaining onion, celery, and mushrooms in the olive oil over medium heat. Add the tomato soup, water, and chopped parsley.
- Pour the topping over the cabbage rolls, cover, and bake for 1 hour and 15 minutes.

Makes 10 cabbage rolls.

Nutrition Information per Serving	
Calories	220.42
Protein	15.49 g
Carbs	12.15 g
Fat	12.54 g
Fiber	2.55 g
Net carb	9.60 g

Cajun Pepper Steak

1–1¼ pounds sirloin steak, ½"–1" thick
1 teaspoon Cajun or Creole seasoning
1 tablespoon olive oil
1 medium sweet onion, minced
1 medium green pepper, minced
3 garlic cloves, minced
1½ cups beef broth
1½ cups diced canned tomatoes
2 teaspoons balsamic vinegar
½ teaspoon dried basil
½ teaspoon freshly ground pepper
¼ teaspoon salt
6 cups sliced cabbage
1 tablespoon cornstarch
2 tablespoons water

• Cut steak into thin slices, approximately 1–2" in length. Sprinkle with the Cajun or Creole seasoning mix. (This is a blend of peppers and other spices used in southern cuisine. You should be able to find these in the spice section of your grocery store.)
• Heat the olive oil in a large skillet or stew pot. Add the beef strips and brown on all sides. Add the green pepper, garlic, and onion and sauté for 3–5 minutes or until tender.
• Add the beef broth, canned tomatoes, balsamic vinegar, and spices to the beef and vegetables. Cover, reduce heat, and simmer for 45 minutes.

continued

- Cut the cabbage into long strips about a ¼″ thick. The cabbage will take the place of mashed potatoes served in the south with this dish. Bring a large pot of water to a boil just 5 minutes before serving. Put the cabbage in the pot and cook for 3–5 minutes. You want the cabbage to be a little firm.
- While the cabbage is cooking, whisk the cornstarch into the water and add to the beef mixture. Cook, stirring constantly, until the sauce is thickened.
- Drain the cabbage well. Serve the beef over the hot cabbage.

Makes 4 servings.

Nutrition Information per Serving

Calories	327.13
Protein	33.30 g
Carbs	15.25 g
Fat	14.81 g
Fiber	5.11 g
Net carb	10.14 g

Chili

••••••••••

1½ pounds ground round
1 tablespoon olive oil
1 large sweet onion, minced
1 green pepper, minced
28-fluid-ounce can diced tomatoes
10-fluid-ounce can kidney beans
10½-ounce can tomato soup
1 teaspoon cayenne
salt & freshly ground pepper, to taste

• Preheat oven to 350°.
• In a heavy skillet, heat olive oil over medium heat and add ground round. Add salt & pepper to taste and cook, stirring to break up the meat into bite-sized pieces, until completely browned, approximately 5 minutes. Using a slotted spoon, remove the meat from the skillet and place in a 4-quart casserole dish.
• Place onions and green pepper in the skillet and sauté until soft, about 5 minutes. Using slotted spoon, remove from skillet and add to casserole dish.
• Add cayenne, tomatoes, kidney beans, and tomato soup to the casserole dish and stir until well mixed.
• Place casserole dish in oven and bake for at least 1 hour and up to 3 hours. If baking for more than 1 hour, reduce heat and stir every hour or so to combine and keep from sticking. This tastes better the longer it simmers.
Makes 6 servings.

NOTE: This recipe has reduced amounts of kidney beans to keep the carb content reasonable. Best served with a green salad.

Nutrition Information per Serving	
Calories	310.35
Protein	26.11 g
Carbs	18.76 g
Fat	16.75 g
Fiber	4.39 g
Net carb	14.37 g

Green Bean Chili

1½ pounds ground round
1 tablespoon olive oil
1 large sweet onion, minced
1 green pepper, minced
28-fluid-ounce can diced
  tomatoes
10.5-ounce can tomato soup

2 cups green beans, cut into ½"
  pieces
2–3 tablespoons tomato paste
1 teaspoon cayenne
salt & freshly ground pepper,
  to taste

- Preheat oven to 350°.
- In a heavy skillet, heat olive oil over medium heat and add the meat. Add salt & pepper to taste and cook, stirring to break up the meat into bite-sized pieces, until completely browned, approximately 5 minutes. Using slotted spoon, remove the meat from the skillet and place in an ovenproof casserole dish or Dutch oven.
- Place onions and green pepper in the skillet and sauté until soft, about 5 minutes. Using the slotted spoon, remove from skillet and add to baking dish.
- Add cayenne, tomatoes, cut-up green beans, tomato paste, and tomato soup and stir until well mixed.
- Place baking dish in the oven and bake for at least 1 hour and up to 3 hours. If baking for a longer period, reduce heat and stir every hour or so to combine and keep from sticking.

Makes 6 servings.

TIP: This chili freezes well and is a bit spicier the next time around.

Thanks to Nancy Shumacher of Lutz, Florida, for the idea of using green beans.

Nutrition Information per Serving

Calories	325.3
Protein	24.57 g
Carbs	18.42 g
Fat	17.31 g
Fiber	3.62 g
Net carb	14.80 g

Grilled Dijon Pork Chops

4 loin pork chops, 1½″ thick & bone in

4 tablespoons Dijon mustard

6 teaspoons olive oil

1 clove garlic, minced

½ teaspoon dried rosemary

1 teaspoon dried thyme

1 teaspoon freshly ground pepper

½ teaspoon salt

• Combine mustard, olive oil, herbs, and salt & pepper in a small bowl. Pour mixture over chops in a shallow bowl and turn to coat. Let stand for 15–20 minutes.
• Preheat grill to medium high. Add the pork chops, close the lid, and grill, turning once, for 5–6 minutes a side or until juice runs clear and meat is cooked through. Test for doneness before removing from grill.
Makes 4 servings.

Nutrition Information per Serving	
Calories	389.11
Protein	23.26 g
Carbs	0.46 g
Fat	32.78 g
Fiber	0.14 g
Net carb	0.32 g

Grilled Herb Steak

2 pounds boneless sirloin steak (1½″ thick)
½ cup red wine
2 tablespoons olive oil
½ teaspoon dried rosemary
1 teaspoon dried thyme
1 teaspoon freshly ground pepper
½ teaspoon salt

- Place the steak in a shallow dish. In a small bowl, whisk together the olive oil, red wine, thyme, rosemary, and salt & pepper. Pour over steak and turn to coat. Cover and refrigerate for 1–2 hours.
- Heat grill to medium high. Place steak on grill and close cover. Grill for 8–10 minutes a side for medium, depending on thickness of steak. Test for doneness by making a small cut in the center of the steak.
- Transfer steak to cutting board and tent with foil for 5 minutes. Slice thinly across the grain.

Makes 6–8 servings.

Nutrition Information per Serving

Calories	375.05
Protein	28.47 g
Carbs	0.88 g
Fat	26.50 g
Fiber	0.14 g
Net carb	0.74 g

Grilled Pork Chops
with White Wine

4 loin pork chops (about 1½ pounds with bone in)
¼ cup white wine
½ cup fresh lemon juice
¼ cup olive oil
2 tablespoons fresh parsley, chopped
2 tablespoons fresh rosemary, chopped
2 tablespoons finely minced onion
1 tablespoon freshly ground pepper

• Combine all ingredients in a shallow pan. Add pork chops and turn to coat. Let stand for half an hour to an hour in the fridge.
• Preheat grill to medium heat. Add chops and grill for 5–6 minutes a side depending on thickness. Check doneness by making a small cut in the middle of the chop.
Makes 4 servings.

**Nutrition Information
per Serving**

Calories	348.74
Protein	23.46 g
Carbs	3.59 g
Fat	25.84 g
Fiber	0.47 g
Net carb	3.12 g

Grilled Sirloin with Red Wine Sauce

2 pounds sirloin steak, 1½" thick
2 tablespoons freshly ground pepper
1 teaspoon salt
Red Wine Steak Sauce (see recipe)

- Preheat grill to medium high.
- Dust steak with salt & pepper and rub into skin.
- Grill 8–9 minutes on each side for medium or until desired doneness. Test with a small knife before removing from grill.
- Remove to carving board and tent with tinfoil for 5 minutes. Slice the steak on the diagonal into thin slices and pour the Red Wine Steak Sauce over individual servings.

Makes 8 servings.

Nutrition Information per Serving

Calories	278.39
Protein	21.59 g
Carbs	1.85 g
Fat	19.27 g
Fiber	0.24 g
Net carb	1.61 g

Grilled Tenderloin
with Fresh Herb Salsa

4 tenderloin steaks (6 ounces), 1½″ thick
1 tablespoon olive oil
1 tablespoon freshly ground pepper
salt, to taste
4 slices bacon
kitchen string
Fresh Herb Salsa (see recipe)

• Wrap each steak with a piece of bacon and secure with kitchen string, making steaks uniform in size.
• Rub steaks with olive oil and pepper. Salt to taste.
• Grill over hot BBQ until desired doneness (generally 6–8 minutes per side for rare, 8–10 minutes per side for medium, and 10–12 minutes per side for well done). The cooking time will vary with the thickness of your steak.
• Place on a serving platter, cut off the string, and let sit for 3–4 minutes. Serve with a hefty dollop of Fresh Herb Salsa on each steak.
Makes 4 servings.

Nutrition Information per Serving

Calories	370.57
Protein	14.02 g
Carbs	1.53 g
Fat	35.72 g
Fiber	0.16 g
Net carb	1.37 g

Ham & Cheese Roll-Up

1 leaf green lettuce
1 slice ham
1 slice processed cheese
1 tablespoon either mustard or mayonnaise

• Spread the mustard or mayonnaise over the lettuce leaf. Line with the ham and then the cheese slice. Roll up the lettuce leaf, tucking in any stray edges. Wrap in waxed paper and twist the ends to make a secure seal.

NOTE: These make a great little snack and can be carried to work or play (e.g., the golf course). They are also a great breakfast alternative. You can add some cut-up veggies for variety and extra flavor. These are the lowest-carb wraps you can make.

Nutrition Information per Serving	
Calories	208.20
Protein	11.54 g
Carbs	1.77 g
Fat	17.25 g
Fiber	0.11 g
Net carb	1.66 g

Lamb Chops with Herbs

¼ cup white wine vinegar

1 tablespoon chopped fresh rosemary

1 tablespoon chopped fresh thyme

1 clove garlic, minced

1 tablespoon olive oil

salt & freshly ground pepper, to taste

8 loin lamb chops

• In a shallow bowl, mix all ingredients except the lamb chops. Add chops and let stand at room temperature for 5–10 minutes, turning to coat.

• Preheat grill to medium high. Place the chops on the BBQ and grill, turning once, for approximately 5–7 minutes a side for medium chops. Check for doneness before removing from grill.

Makes 4 servings.

Nutrition Information per Serving	
Calories	225.18
Protein	27.31 g
Carbs	1.11 g
Fat	11.34 g
Fiber	0.21 g
Net carb	0.90 g

Lemon Herb Lamb Chops

8 lean lamb chops, about 1½″ thick
Lemon Herb Marinade for Pork (see recipe)

• Place chops in a shallow dish and pour marinade over them, turning to coat. Let stand 1 hour at room temperature.
• Preheat oven broiler. Spray broiler rack with a nonstick agent and place chops on rack. Place rack in oven about 6″ from broiler. Broil for approximately 7–8 minutes on each side, until well browned for medium to well done. Doneness will vary with thickness, so always test before removing from oven. *Makes 4 servings.*

Nutrition Information per Serving

Calories	293.06
Protein	20.78 g
Carbs	2.21 g
Fat	21.45 g
Fiber	0.31 g
Net carb	1.90 g

London Broil

....

1½ pounds boneless sirloin steak (1½" thick)

⅔ cup soy sauce

3 tablespoons Worcestershire Sauce

2 cloves garlic, minced

1 teaspoon dried thyme

1 teaspoon freshly ground pepper

- Place steak in a shallow dish. In a small bowl, whisk together the soy sauce, Worcestershire Sauce, garlic, pepper, and thyme. Pour over steak and turn to coat. Cover and refrigerate for 2–4 hours.
- Heat grill to medium high. Place steak on grill and close cover. Grill for 8–10 minutes a side for medium, depending on thickness of steak. Test for doneness by making a small cut in the center of the steak.
- Transfer steak to cutting board and tent with foil for 5 minutes. Slice thinly across the grain.

Makes 4–6 servings.

Nutrition Information per Serving	
Calories	380.78
Protein	34.72 g
Carbs	1.72 g
Fat	24.56 g
Fiber	0.16 g
Net carb	1.56 g

Meat Loaf

1½ pounds lean ground beef
1 celery stalk, diced
½ medium red onion, diced
2 small fresh mushrooms, diced
1 egg, slightly beaten
1 tablespoon fine bread crumbs
3 tablespoons undiluted beef consommé
1 teaspoon Fine Herbs
salt & freshly ground pepper, to taste

- Preheat oven to 400°.
- Put meat in a large mixing bowl and add all the other ingredients but beef consommé. Mix well with wooden spoon.
- Place in a loaf pan sprayed with a nonstick agent. Press firmly into pan with spoon and smooth top. Spoon beef consommé on top of mixture.
- Bake for one hour.

Makes 6 servings.

Nutrition Information per Serving

Calories	251.34
Protein	23.08 g
Carbs	4.64 g
Fat	15.13 g
Fiber	0.37 g
Net carb	4.27 g

Meat Loaf with Tomato Sauce

1½ pounds lean ground beef
1 celery stalk, diced
½ medium red onion, diced
2 small fresh mushrooms, diced
1 egg, slightly beaten
1 tablespoon fine bread crumbs
salt & freshly ground pepper, to taste

Tomato Sauce
4 tablespoons tomato paste
1 tablespoon olive oil
2 tablespoons water
1 teaspoon Fine Herbs

- Preheat oven to 400°.
- Put meat in a large mixing bowl and add all the other ingredients but tomato sauce. Mix well with a wooden spoon.
- Place in a loaf pan sprayed with a nonstick agent. Press firmly into pan with spoon and smooth top.
- Mix tomato paste, water, and olive oil to make sauce and spoon over mixture. Sprinkle with Fine Herbs.
- Bake for 1 hour.

Makes 6 servings.

NOTE: Serve either Meat Loaf recipe with Creamy Garlic Cauliflower for what looks like a meat-and-potatoes standard.

Nutrition Information per Serving

Calories	237.28
Protein	22.53 g
Carbs	4.08 g
Fat	14.04 g
Fiber	0.61 g
Net carb	3.47 g

Oven-Baked Beef Stew

2 pounds trimmed stewing beef
1 tablespoon olive oil
6 carrots
2 cups cubed turnip
6 small onions
6 large celery stalks, including leafy tops
12–18 mushrooms
2 tablespoons flour
1 teaspoon cornstarch
1 teaspoon Fine Herbs
½ teaspoon salt
1 teaspoon ground black pepper

- At least 3½ hours before serving, preheat oven to 350°.
- Trim all visible fat off meat and cut into ½″ pieces. Mix together ground pepper, salt, and Fine Herbs. Sprinkle spices on meat and toss to coat.
- Wash all vegetables and cut carrots and turnip into bite-sized pieces. If the onions are very large, cut them into quarters. Put carrots, turnip, and onion into a large bowl of cold water and set aside. Cut the celery into 2″ pieces and set aside with the whole mushrooms. Save the leafy tops of the celery.
- In a large stew pot, heat olive oil over medium heat. Brown the meat on all sides. When the meat has been browned, add enough cold water to cover the meat. Scrape any brown bits off the bottom of the pot into the water. Drain and add the carrots, turnip, onion, and leafy celery tops to the pot. Make sure that the water covers the vegetables.

continued

- Cover and bake at 350° for 2 hours, stirring once in a while.
- Remove pot from the oven. Remove any remnants of the leafy celery tops from the stew. (These add great flavor and are often completely incorporated by this time.)
- Turn the oven to 400°. Add the celery sticks and mushrooms to the stew. Make sure that there is sufficient water to cover the vegetables.
- Mix 2 tablespoons of flour with 1 teaspoon of cornstarch in a small bowl. Add hot liquid from the stew a bit at a time to dissolve the flour and cornstarch until you have a very smooth thin liquid. Add this liquid to the stew pot and stir well. This will help the sauce to thicken during the last hour of baking.
- Cover the stew pot and place back in the oven for an hour.
- Serve in large bowls.

Makes 6 servings.

VARIATION: You can add other vegetables to the stew. If you add more delicate vegetables, such as asparagus or green beans, do not add them until the last hour of baking.

Nutrition Information per Serving

Calories	288.17
Protein	30.07 g
Carbs	20.38 g
Fat	9.69 g
Fiber	5.94 g
Net carb	14.44 g

Peppered Steak

1 steak, 2–3 pounds (tenderloin, sirloin, or New York strip,
   at least 1½″ thick)
2 tablespoons olive oil
2 garlic cloves, finely minced
1½ teaspoons cracked pepper
½ teaspoon cayenne pepper
½ teaspoon dried thyme leaves
½ teaspoon dried oregano

- Preheat oven to 450° or preheat grill to medium high.
- Brush both sides of the steak with the olive oil. Put the peppers, garlic, and spices in a small bowl and mix to blend. Spread the mixture evenly on both sides of the steak and rub into the meat. Let stand for 20 minutes.
- If baking in the oven, bake for 5 minutes, reduce temperature to 375°, and continue baking for another 25–30 minutes for medium or until desired doneness. Check for doneness before removing from oven.
- If grilling, cook on medium-high grill, turning occasionally, for 18–20 minutes for medium or until desired doneness. Check for doneness before removing from grill.
- Place steak on cutting board and tent with foil for 5 minutes. Cut on the diagonal into thin slices.

Makes 8 servings.

Nutrition Information per Serving

Calories	362.35
Protein	28.47 g
Carbs	0.73 g
Fat	26.50 g
Fiber	0.16 g
Net carb	0.57 g

Pork Loin in White Wine

4 boneless loin chops (1 pound)
1 teaspoon freshly ground pepper
1 tablespoon olive oil
1 tablespoon chopped fresh rosemary
½ cup chicken bouillon
1 cup fresh mushrooms, sliced
½ cup white wine
1 teaspoon lime zest
1 tablespoon lime juice
1 teaspoon cornstarch
1 tablespoon chopped fresh parsley
1 clove garlic, minced

• Heat oil in frying pan over medium heat. Grind pepper over chops and press in. Brown chops in oil, 2–3 minutes a side. Transfer to ovenproof pan and put in a warm oven (300°).
• Add garlic and mushrooms to pan and sauté for 3–4 minutes, until soft. Add bouillon, wine, lime zest, juice, and fresh rosemary to pan and bring to a boil. If the sauce is a bit thin, dissolve the cornstarch in a little water and add it to the mixture.
• Add chops back to the pan and simmer over medium heat, turning to coat for 3–4 minutes. Serve chops with sauce and a sprinkle of fresh parsley.
Makes 4 servings.

Nutrition Information per Serving

Calories	270.13
Protein	24.02 g
Carbs	2.54 g
Fat	15.53 g
Fiber	0.52 g
Net carb	2.02 g

Pork Medallions with Cream Sauce

1½ pounds pork tenderloin
1 tablespoon butter
1 tablespoon olive oil
3 green onions, chopped
1 cup sliced fresh mushrooms
½ cup heavy cream

½ cup chicken bouillon
1 tablespoon white wine
½ teaspoon cornstarch
salt & freshly ground pepper,
 to taste

- Cut pork tenderloin crosswise into 1″ thick medallions. Sprinkle with salt & freshly ground pepper.
- Heat butter and olive oil in a heavy frying pan over medium-high heat.
- Working in batches, sauté medallions until browned on both sides and cooked through, about 4 minutes a side. Transfer medallions to ovenproof dish, tent with foil, and place in a warm oven (about 250°).
- Add mushrooms and green onion to pan and sauté until soft, about 3 minutes. Add cream, chicken bouillon, and wine. Bring mixture to a boil and lower heat. Cook, stirring constantly, until thick enough to coat spoon. You may need to add the cornstarch to help thicken. If cornstarch is needed, dissolve in a small amount of water before adding to the sauce.
- Season sauce with salt & freshly ground pepper. Return the medallions to the pan and continue cooking for 2 minutes while stirring constantly to coat.
- Divide warm medallions onto four plates and cover with sauce.

Makes 4 servings.

Nutrition Information per Serving	
Calories	409.49
Protein	35.43 g
Carbs	2.95 g
Fat	27.58 g
Fiber	0.36 g
Net carb	2.59 g

Pork Stir-Fry

2 tablespoons olive oil
2 cups diced cooked pork
½ cup onion, quartered and thinly sliced
1 cup sliced mushrooms
1 cup diced celery
2 cups chopped bok choy
2 cups zucchini, cut in half and thinly sliced
6 cups cabbage, thinly sliced
Oriental Stir-Fry Sauce (see recipe)

- Heat olive oil in a heavy frying pan over medium heat.
- Add the cubed, cooked pork with the onion and sauté 3–4 minutes.
- Add the zucchini, celery, and bok choy and continue cooking until all vegetables are just done. This will take 4–5 minutes. Stir in Oriental Stir-Fry Sauce and continue cooking for another few minutes until sauce is bubbling.
- While the stir-fry is cooking, steam the sliced cabbage until just done but still firm. This will take 4 or 5 minutes.
- Evenly divide the steamed cabbage on 4 plates. Spoon the stir-fry on top of the cabbage and garnish with sesame seeds.

Makes 4 servings.

NOTE: This is a really tasty way to use up any leftover pork roast or even chops.

Nutrition Information per Serving

Calories	377.85
Protein	24.19 g
Carbs	20.34 g
Fat	24.06 g
Fiber	8.17 g
Net carb	12.17 g

Pot Roast

3–4 pound boneless rump or shoulder roast

3 tablespoons olive oil

1 tablespoon butter

3 sweet onions, cut into 8ths

1 tablespoon paprika

½ teaspoon Fine Herbs

½ teaspoon dried thyme leaves

½ teaspoon dried oregano leaves

3 garlic cloves, crushed

3 leafy celery tops

3 bay leaves

2 cups beef broth

3 tablespoons red wine vinegar (or balsamic vinegar)

½ teaspoon freshly ground pepper

¼ teaspoon salt

6–8 carrots cut into 1½" pieces

1 medium turnip cut into 1½" pieces

1 tablespoon flour

1 teaspoon cornstarch

- Preheat oven to 300°.
- Spray large Dutch oven or covered roasting pan with a nonstick cooking spray. Heat olive oil and butter in the roasting pan over medium-high heat on the stove-top. Salt & pepper the roast and brown on all sides. Remove the roast from pan and set aside.

continued

- Reduce the heat to medium, add the onions to the pan, and sauté for 5 minutes. Add the garlic, Fine Herbs, paprika, oregano, and thyme and continue cooking for 1 minute.
- Add the beef broth and vinegar and bring to a boil. Add the meat back in, then the carrots, turnip, bay leaves, and celery tops. You want to almost, but not completely, cover the vegetables with liquid.
- Cover and place in the oven to cook for 2 hours. After 2 hours, remove the celery tops, turn the roast, and return to the oven for 1 more hour. If there is not sufficient liquid to almost cover the vegetables, add a little extra beef broth. This is not a stew, so it is important to leave some of the vegetables poking out of the liquid so that they caramelize in the oven. At this point, you can add some additional vegetables for variety if desired. Vegetables that blend well with the flavors include mushrooms and asparagus.
- Remove the pan from the oven. Place the meat on a platter and cover with foil. Place the vegetables around the meat for presentation or in a separate serving bowl.
- Mix the tablespoon of flour and teaspoon of cornstarch with a little water in a small dish until they are completely blended and you have a thin liquid. Place the roasting pan on a stove-top element and bring heat to medium. Add the flour and cornstarch and bring the mixture to a boil, stirring constantly until thickened.
- Carve the roast into slices and serve with vegetables and sauce.

Makes 6–8 servings due to shrinkage of the meat.

NOTE: This is a really delicious roast that is moist and full of flavor. It is one of our favorites. It can be kept in the fridge and reheated in a day or two. It also makes a wonderful lunch meal the next day.

NOTE: You can add some squash as a vegetable variation with the other vegetables at the beginning. I might also add mushrooms, green beans, or asparagus during the last hour of baking for additional flavor and color. The carb content will increase slightly with these additional vegetables.

Nutrition Information per Serving	
Calories	391.52
Protein	39.12 g
Carbs	10.41 g
Fat	20.28 g
Fiber	3.01 g
Net carb	7.40 g

Quick Beef Hash

....

2 cups leftover beef cut into bite-sized pieces
1 cup sliced fresh mushrooms
1 cup diced red onion
2 tablespoons olive oil
salt & freshly ground pepper, to taste

- Heat oil in a frying pan over medium heat. Add all ingredients and seasonings. Cook, turning frequently, until onions and mushrooms are soft, about 5–6 minutes.
Makes 2 servings.

TIP: This is a really good, quick lunch and can be made with leftover steak or roast beef.

Nutrition Information per Serving	
Calories	293.25
Protein	16.91 g
Carbs	7.64 g
Fat	22.35 g
Fiber	1.56 g
Net carb	6.08 g

Rack of Lamb with Herbs & Spices

2 racks of lamb (1½–2 pounds)
1 tablespoon olive oil
1½ tablespoons Dijon mustard
1 teaspoon dried rosemary
1 teaspoon Fine Herbs
salt & freshly ground pepper to taste
Dijon Herb Sauce (see recipe)

- Preheat oven to 450°.
- Spray a roasting rack and a large roasting pan with a nonstick spray.
- Pat racks of lamb dry.
- Heat the olive oil in a large frying pan. Brown the racks of lamb on all sides, about 2–3 minutes a side. You may have to brown racks one at a time depending on size, and you may need to add olive oil if browning separately.
- Remove lamb to a rack in a roasting pan. Brush lamb with mustard on both sides and sprinkle with rosemary, Fine Herbs, and salt & pepper.
- Roast at 450° for about 15–20 minutes for medium or until desired doneness. Roasting time will vary with thickness of rack. Check doneness by making a small cut in the meat.
- Transfer meat to a serving platter, tent with foil, and let stand for 5 minutes. Cut racks into two servings each and garnish with sprigs of fresh rosemary. Serve with Dijon Herb Sauce. *Makes 4 servings.*

NOTE: These racks of lamb may also be grilled on a medium-high grill for approximately the same amount of time.

Nutrition Information per Serving	
Calories	426.28
Protein	21.14 g
Carbs	2.46 g
Fat	35.66 g
Fiber	0.42 g
Net carb	2.04 g

Roast Beef
with Creamy Red Wine Sauce

3–4 pound prime rib roast (or any preferred cut)
2 tablespoons Dijon mustard
½ tablespoon olive oil
1 teaspoon each dried rosemary & thyme
¼ teaspoon allspice
Creamy Red Wine Sauce (see recipe)

• In a small dish, whisk together Dijon mustard, oil, and spices. Place roast in a roasting pan treated with a nonstick agent. Brush roast with the mustard-herb preparation and let stand for 30 minutes at room temperature.
• Preheat oven to 350°. Place roast in oven and cook for approximately 25–30 minutes a pound for medium. Remove roast to a carving board, tent with foil, and let sit for 5 minutes before carving. Serve with Creamy Red Wine Sauce. *Makes 6–8 servings.*

Nutrition Information per Serving	
Calories	274.27
Protein	33.31 g
Carbs	1.48 g
Fat	12.57 g
Fiber	0.17 g
Net carb	1.31 g

Roast Leg of Lamb

3–4 pound leg of lamb
½ tablespoon olive oil
½ teaspoon dried rosemary leaves
¼ teaspoon dried thyme leaves
½ teaspoon ground black pepper
¼ teaspoon salt
2 tablespoons flour
1 teaspoon cornstarch

- Preheat oven to 400°.
- Brush roast with the olive oil. Mix the dried herbs together and sprinkle on the roast. Press herbs into meat with hands.
- Place the roast in a roasting pan and put in the hot oven for 10 minutes to sear the meat and seal in the juices. Turn oven back to 350°. Roast for 45 minutes per pound to allow for the leg bone.
- Remove from oven and let sit for 10 minutes before carving.
- While roast sits, mix the flour and cornstarch into ½ cup of water. Remove all but about a tablespoon of fat from the roasting pan. While stirring constantly, add water mixture to drippings in pan and cook over medium heat until boiling. You may need to add some extra water if the gravy gets too thick. You may also want to add some ground pepper, salt, and Fine Herbs to flavor the gravy.

Makes 6–8 servings, depending on the size of the bone.

NOTE: The nutrition information is calculated using 8 servings.

Nutrition Information per Serving	
Calories	306.82
Protein	35.88 g
Carbs	1.86 g
Fat	16.12 g
Fiber	0.15 g
Net carb	1.71 g

Savory Pork Chops with Gravy

4 loin pork chops, 1½″ thick and bone in

2 teaspoons flour

1 tablespoon olive oil

¾ teaspoon dried oregano

¾ teaspoon dried rosemary

1 teaspoon freshly ground pepper

½ teaspoon salt

1 small onion, thinly sliced and separated into rings

1 cup chicken bouillon

• Combine herbs and salt & pepper in a small bowl. Sprinkle herbs over chops and press in with hands.

• In a large nonstick frying pan, heat oil over medium-high heat. Brown chops in oil, for 3–5 minutes on each side, until golden. Remove chops to ovenproof dish and place in a warm oven, approximately 300°.

• Place onion in frying pan and cook for 3–4 minutes until golden. Add the flour, stirring constantly until well blended. Add the chicken bouillon, stirring constantly, and reduce heat to medium. Bring to a boil and continue cooking until the mixture is reduced by half.

• Add the pork chops and any liquid in the pan back to the frying pan and turn to coat. Simmer for 2–3 minutes.

Makes 4 servings.

Nutrition Information per Serving	
Calories	257.64
Protein	24.13 g
Carbs	3.39 g
Fat	15.90 g
Fiber	0.68 g
Net carb	2.71 g

Shepherd's Pie

Creamy Garlic Cauliflower (see recipe)
1½ pounds lean ground beef
½ medium-sized onion, minced
2 cloves garlic, minced
1 teaspoon olive oil
2 tablespoons tomato paste
2 teaspoons Dijon mustard
2 tablespoons water
1 pound green or yellow snap beans
salt & freshly ground pepper, to taste
chopped fresh parsley

- Prepare the Creamy Garlic Cauliflower recipe and set aside.
- Preheat oven to 375°.
- Spray a 3-liter baking dish with a nonstick agent.
- Place the ground beef in a nonstick frying pan, season with freshly ground pepper, and sauté until browned on all sides. This will take 5 or 6 minutes. Break the beef into bite-sized pieces while it is browning.
- Add the onion and garlic to the pan and continue cooking for 3 or 4 minutes, until the onion is soft. Pour or spoon off any fat.
- While the onion is cooking, mix the tomato paste, Dijon mustard, and water in a small dish. Whisk to blend.
- Add the tomato mixture to the beef and continue to cook for 2 minutes while stirring constantly to coat the meat with the sauce. Put the beef into the bottom of the baking dish.

continued

- Wash, trim, and cut the beans into ½″ pieces. Place in water and microwave for 4 minutes. Drain well.
- Place the beans as a layer over the meat. Cover the beans with the Creamy Garlic Cauliflower and sprinkle with some chopped fresh parsley and freshly ground pepper.
- Bake uncovered for 30–40 minutes, until the edges are brown.

Makes 6 servings.

VARIATION: For a slightly sophisticated variation, substitute asparagus spears cut into pieces for the beans. You may also add grated cheese to the topping before baking.

Nutrition Information per Serving

Calories	322.55
Protein	23.52 g
Carbs	7.33 g
Fat	22.22 g
Fiber	1.39 g
Net carb	5.94 g

Steak with Roasted Vegetables

1½-pound sirloin steak, about 2″ thick

2 medium carrots

2 small turnips

1 medium zucchini

8 pearl onions or 1 medium sweet onion

4 tablespoons olive oil

salt & freshly ground pepper, to taste

Dijon Steak Sauce

⅔ cup Dijon mustard

1 teaspoon chopped fresh mint

1 teaspoon chopped fresh thyme

- Preheat oven to 450°.
- Wash and peel carrots. Cut in half lengthwise, then into 1½″ pieces. Wash and peel turnips and cut into 1½″ pieces.
- If using a medium sweet onion, peel and cut into 8ths. If using pearl onions, peel and wash.
- Wash zucchini and cut in half lengthwise, then into 2″ pieces.
- Combine vegetables in a large bowl with 3 tablespoons of olive oil and toss to coat. Sprinkle with freshly ground pepper & salt.
- Spray a large baking pan with a nonstick product and spoon the vegetables into pan. Roast vegetables for 30–40 minutes or until cooked to desired softness, stirring regularly to brown evenly on all sides.

continued

- Brush steak with remaining tablespoon of olive oil. Coat generously with freshly ground pepper & salt. Place steak on a separate small roasting pan prepared with a nonstick product.
- Roast steak until desired doneness, about 30 minutes for medium. Test for doneness by making a small incision in the center of the steak.
- Remove from oven and let stand under a tent of foil for 3–5 minutes. Cut steak into thin strips on the diagonal.
- Mix mustard with the fresh herbs to make sauce. Let stand for at least 30 minutes to allow flavors to blend.
- Serve thinly sliced steak with roasted vegetables and a dollop of mustard sauce.

Makes 4–6 servings.

NOTE: Nutrition information is calculated using 4 servings.

Nutrition Information per Serving	
Calories	559.63
Protein	37.83 g
Carbs	17.87 g
Fat	42.86 g
Fiber	4.00 g
Net carb	13.87 g

Sweet & Sour Chops

4 pork loin chops
¾ cup chicken broth
4 packets Splenda
2 tablespoons white wine vinegar
2 cloves garlic, minced
½ teaspoon ground black pepper
1 teaspoon cornstarch

• Heat olive oil in a large frying pan and brown chops on both sides. Cook until almost done, about 4–5 minutes a side. Remove from pan, place in an ovenproof dish, and place in a warm (250°) oven.
• Add chicken stock, Splenda, white wine vinegar, garlic, and pepper to frying pan. Stir to blend well. In a small bowl, add a bit of the liquid to 1 teaspoon of cornstarch to dissolve. Add this liquid to the pan and bring to a boil. Cook, stirring constantly, until thick and bubbly. This will take about 3–5 minutes.
• Return chops to the frying pan, adding any juices from the roasting pan. Turn to coat and stir to blend all juices.
Makes 4 servings.

Nutrition Information per Serving	
Calories	280.17
Protein	18.71 g
Carbs	2.42 g
Fat	21.51 g
Fiber	0.11 g
Net carb	2.31 g

Tenderloin of Pork with White Wine

1½ pounds boneless loin of
    pork
2 cloves garlic, quartered
8 slices bacon
2 tablespoons olive oil
1 large onion, cut into 8ths
8 large mushrooms

1 cup chicken bouillon
2 sprigs fresh thyme
2 sprigs fresh rosemary
1 bay leaf
½ cup white wine
salt & freshly ground pepper

- Preheat oven to 350°.
- With a sharp knife, make small openings in the pork loin and insert garlic. Season pork with salt & freshly ground pepper. Wrap each pork tenderloin in bacon lengthways. Tie with kitchen string in 2 or 3 places to secure the bacon.
- Heat the oil until hot in a 2-quart casserole dish. Add the pork and sauté until golden brown on all sides, about 6–7 minutes. Remove and set aside.
- Add onions and mushrooms and sauté until golden. Return the meat to the casserole dish. Add chicken bouillon, thyme, rosemary, and bay leaf and bring to a boil over medium heat.
- Cover and place in the oven for 1½ hours. Add the white wine to the casserole dish 30 minutes before serving and return to the oven.
- Remove the casserole dish from the oven. Remove the pork tenderloins and cut off the kitchen string. Cut into slices, using a sharp knife to make diagonal cuts. Serve with onion, mushrooms, and a little sauce.

Makes 4 servings.

Nutrition Information per Serving	
Calories	565.58
Protein	39.13 g
Carbs	5.43 g
Fat	39.50 g
Fiber	1.17 g
Net carb	4.26 g

Teriyaki Burgers

1 pound lean ground beef

Marinade:
¼ cup soy sauce
¼ cup minced red onion
½ teaspoon grated fresh ginger (¼ teaspoon dried ginger)
1 clove garlic, minced
½ teaspoon ground cumin
freshly ground pepper, to taste

• Combine soy sauce, onions, garlic, ginger, and pepper in a small bowl.
• Add soy mixture to beef and mix thoroughly. Divide into four portions and form patties.
• Preheat grill to medium high and cook 4–5 minutes a side, depending on the thickness of the patty. Burgers should be cooked through.
Makes 4 servings.

TIP: This marinade is also good with pork chops or chicken breasts.

Nutrition Information per Serving	
Calories	336.59
Protein	34.27 g
Carbs	1.89 g
Fat	20.16 g
Fiber	0.28 g
Net carb	1.61 g

COOKIES

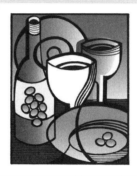

Almond Cookies

2 cups ground almonds
½ cup granular Splenda
¼ cup soy flour
2 teaspoons vanilla extract
½ teaspoon almond extract
2 egg whites
2 tablespoons melted butter

- Preheat oven to 350°.
- Whisk the egg whites until frothy. Add the vanilla and almond extracts and set aside.
- Combine the ground almonds, soy flour, and Splenda in a bowl and mix well. Add the egg white mixture and blend. Slowly add the melted butter, stirring constantly.
- You will have a heavy, sticky dough. Pick up the batter with a teaspoon and use fingers to shape a round, flat cookie about a ¼" thick. Place on a cookie sheet covered with parchment paper. Repeat until all the batter is used.
- Bake for 20–25 minutes until lightly browned all over.

Makes 3 dozen delicious cookies.

NOTE: If you can't find ground almonds (at the health food store or specialty baking store), you can grind your own using blanched almonds and a food processor or blender.

Nutrition Information per Cookie

Calories	41.34
Protein	1.57 g
Carbs	1.67 g
Fat	3.46 g
Fiber	0.73 g
Net carb	0.94 g

Almond Peanut Butter Cookies

⅓ cup vanilla whey protein

⅓ cup ground almond

½ teaspoon baking soda

8 packets Splenda

⅓ cup soy flour

½ teaspoon baking powder

1 teaspoon xanthan gum

1 cup peanut butter, chunky or smooth

2 eggs

¼ cup olive oil

1 teaspoon vanilla extract

⅓ cup water

- Preheat oven to 350°.
- Mix all dry ingredients in a large bowl and blend well with a wooden spoon.
- Whisk eggs with olive oil in a separate bowl. Add water and vanilla and whisk until blended. Add peanut butter and mix with a fork until completely blended.
- Make a well in the dry ingredients and pour the wet ingredients in the well and stir until fully blended.
- You may either drop by teaspoons or form into small balls and then press with a fork. Place cookies on a cookie sheet lined with parchment paper.
- Bake 10–12 minutes until just brown at the edges.

Makes 4 ½ dozen cookies.

NOTE: You will want to use commercially ground almonds, sometimes called almond meal, for these cookies so that they blend well. These cookies freeze well and thaw within minutes.

Thanks again to my sister Stephanie, who helped me to develop these really delicious cookies.

Nutrition Information per Cookie

Calories	49.38
Protein	2.32 g
Carbs	1.27 g
Fat	4.22 g
Fiber	0.10 g
Net carb	1.17 g

Chocolate Coconut Balls

1 can Eagle Brand Milk
5 cups dessicated coconut (unsweetened & fine)
250 grams Lindt 70% Cocoa Dark Chocolate
12 packets Splenda
½ cup butter

- Melt the butter. Mix the coconut and Splenda in a large bowl. Add the butter and milk and blend well. Cover with plastic wrap and place in fridge for 2–3 hours.
- Melt the chocolate in the top of a double boiler, being careful not to let any moisture get into the chocolate.
- Using a small teaspoon, scoop the coconut mixture into your palm and roll into a small ball. Dip the ball into the melted chocolate using a fork or candy dipper. Let drip to allow excess chocolate to come off, and place on a cookie sheet lined with waxed paper.
(I roll about a dozen at a time, then dip them into the chocolate.)
- When the cookie sheet is full, place flat in your freezer for 15–20 minutes.
Makes 100 chocolate balls.

NOTE: I keep my chocolate balls in an air-tight container in the freezer to keep them extra fresh. They take only a minute to thaw.

These are really delicious treats that I make every year at Christmas. The original recipe came from a good friend, Wanda Murphy, of Victoria, British Columbia.

Nutrition Information per Ball

Calories	66.88
Protein	0.76 g
Carbs	4.30 g
Fat	5.22 g
Fiber	0.93 g
Net carb	3.37 g

Coconut Macaroons

1 egg, beaten

4 packets Splenda

2 cups shredded, sweetened coconut

½ teaspoon vanilla extract

¼ cup heavy cream

- Preheat oven to 325°.
- Put beaten egg into heavy mixing bowl. Add Splenda and mix with a fork. Add vanilla extract and coconut. Finally add the heavy cream and blend well.
- Using a heaping teaspoon of batter, mound into 1″ high mounds on a greased cookie sheet or a sheet lined with parchment or a "sil" baking pad.
- Bake until golden brown, about 10–12 minutes.
- Remove from oven and leave on the cookie sheet for a couple of minutes to cool; then remove to a cake rack to continue cooling.

Makes 18 cookies.

Nutrition Information per Macaroon	
Calories	78.41
Protein	1.35 g
Carbs	5.72 g
Fat	5.95 g
Fiber	0.89 g
Net carb	4.83 g

Crunchy Peanut Butter Cookies

1 cup crunchy peanut butter

½ cup granular Splenda

1 egg

- Preheat oven to 325°.
- Mix all ingredients in a bowl.
- Roll dough into 24 balls. Place balls on cookie sheet covered with parchment paper and flatten with a fork.
- Bake for 12 minutes. Cool before removing from the pan.

Makes 24 cookies.

Thanks to Donna Omeniuk of Winnipeg, Manitoba, for this really great cookie recipe. I think that Donna may have adapted the recipe that appears on the Kraft Peanut Butter jar.

Nutrition Information per Cookie

Calories	71.58
Protein	2.92 g
Carbs	2.54 g
Fat	6.19 g
Fiber	0.00 g
Net carb	2.54 g

Flax Cookies

½ cup butter

12 packets Splenda

1 cup flax seed meal

2 eggs

1 teaspoon vanilla extract

½ cup ground almonds

½ cup oat flour

½ cup rolled oats

½ tablespoon baking soda

1 teaspoon xanthan gum

- In a large bowl, cream butter and Splenda with an electric mixer. Add the flax seed meal and blend.
- In a separate bowl, beat the eggs and vanilla. Add the flax seed mixture and beat on low until thoroughly blended.
- Mix all other dry ingredients in a separate bowl.
- Mix the dry and wet ingredients together.
- Separate dough into two equal portions. Form dough into 2 round logs (1″ in diameter) and cover with plastic wrap. Place in the freezer to chill for 15–20 minutes.
- Preheat oven to 350°.
- Slice the dough into ¼″ thin slices. Place slices on cookie sheet lined with parchment paper.
- Bake for 12–15 minutes, until brown at the edges. Remove to a cookie rack and cool.

Makes 4 dozen cookies.

NOTE: These are really delicious, crunchy cookies that provide great nutrition along with taste.

Nutrition Information per Cookie	
Calories	47.66
Protein	1.45 g
Carbs	2.87 g
Fat	3.97 g
Fiber	1.08 g
Net carb	1.79 g

Icebox Cookies

½ cup oat flour

¼ cup soy flour

¼ cup ground almond

¼ teaspoon baking soda

⅛ teaspoon salt

4 tablespoons butter

⅔ cup granular Splenda

1 teaspoon vanilla extract

1 large egg white

- Combine the flours, ground almonds, baking soda, and salt. Set aside.
- Beat butter at medium speed until light and fluffy, gradually adding Splenda until well blended. Add vanilla and egg white and continue beating until blended.
- Add the flour mixture and stir until combined fully. Turn dough onto a piece of waxed paper and roll into a 6″ log. Put in the freezer for 3 hours or until very firm.
- Preheat oven to 350°.
- Cut the dough log into 24 even slices (approximately ¼″ thick). Place slices 1″ apart on a cooking sheet lined with parchment paper.
- Bake for 8–10 minutes, until the edges and bottoms are just browned. Remove from cookie sheet with a spatula and cool on a wire rack.
Makes 24 cookies.

NOTE: These cookies freeze well and thaw in just minutes.

Nutrition Information per Cookie	
Calories	36.51
Protein	1.04 g
Carbs	2.53 g
Fat	2.84 g
Fiber	0.53 g
Net carb	2.00 g

Maxine's Chocolate Cookies

⅔ cup soy flour

⅓ cup oat flour

⅓ cup ground almonds

8 packets Splenda

1 teaspoon baking powder

1 teaspoon baking soda

1 teaspoon xanthan gum

3 squares unsweetened baking chocolate (3 ounces)

2 eggs

¼ cup olive oil

1 teaspoon vanilla extract

¼ cup heavy cream

½ cup finely shredded zucchini with skin

⅓ cup additional ground almond for finishing

- Mix all dry ingredients in a large bowl and blend well.
- Melt chocolate in the top of a double boiler and then set aside to cool slightly.
- Whisk eggs with olive oil. Add cream, vanilla, and zucchini and whisk to blend.
- Make a well in the dry ingredients, add the egg mixture, and mix well. Add the chocolate and stir until all the chocolate is evenly blended. This will make a heavy, wet batter. Cover with plastic wrap and cool in the fridge for 1 or 2 hours. This makes the batter easier to handle.
- Preheat oven to 325°.

continued

• Using a teaspoon to pick up the batter, roll into small balls in the palms of your hands. Your hands will get sticky, and you will want to wash and dry between batches. Roll the dough balls into the additional ground almonds, forming a thin layer of ground almond. (You may need to knock off any loose almond meal.) Place the balls approximately 1″ apart on a cookie sheet lined with parchment.

• The cookies will flatten while cooking, and the almond coating will crack to show the dark chocolate inside.

• Bake for 10–12 minutes, until browned at the edges.

Makes 4 dozen cookies.

NOTE: These cookies need to be kept in the fridge because of the zucchini in them. They do not keep for very long. They can also be frozen.

This delicious recipe was given to my mother many years ago by a close friend, Maxine Dennis. My sister Stephanie was instrumental in figuring out the low-carb variety.

Nutrition Information per Cookie

Calories	38.13
Protein	1.59 g
Carbs	1.86 g
Fat	3.19 g
Fiber	0.45 g
Net carb	1.41 g

Oatmeal Peanut Butter Cookies

1 cup crunchy peanut butter
½ cup granular Splenda
¼ cup rolled oats
1 egg

- Preheat oven to 325°.
- Mix all ingredients in a bowl. Roll dough into 24 balls.
- Place balls on cookie sheet covered with parchment paper and flatten with a fork.
- Bake for 12 minutes. Cool before removing from the pan.

Makes 24 cookies.

NOTE: Do not use the instant variety of oats since it will dramatically increase the carb content and the glycemic index.

Thanks to Donna Omeniuk of Winnipeg, Manitoba, for the original idea for these cookies.

Nutrition Information per Cookie

Calories	74.68
Protein	3.05 g
Carbs	3.12 g
Fat	6.25 g
Fiber	0.08 g
Net carb	3.04 g

Oatmeal Raisin Cookies

¼ cup flax seed meal

¼ cup sunflower seeds, finely ground

¼ cup pumpkin seeds, finely ground

½ cup ground almonds

½ cup rolled oats (regular oatmeal, not the instant variety)

½ cup soy flour

6 packets Splenda

1 teaspoon cinnamon

1 teaspoon nutmeg

1 teaspoon xanthan gum

2 eggs

3 tablespoons olive oil

½ cup finely shredded zucchini with skin

¼ cup light cream (half & half)

2 teaspoons vanilla extract

¼ cup seedless raisins

- Preheat oven to 350°.
- Mix all dry ingredients in a large bowl and blend well with a wooden spoon.
- Whisk eggs with olive oil in a separate bowl. Add cream and vanilla and whisk until blended. Add shredded zucchini and mix with a fork until completely blended.
- Make a well in the dry ingredients, pour the wet ingredients into the well, and stir until fully blended.
- Drop by teaspoons onto a cookie sheet lined with parchment paper.
- Bake for 10–12 minutes, until just brown at the edges.

Makes 4 ½ dozen cookies.

NOTE: These cookies need to be kept in the fridge or frozen.

Thanks again to my sister Stephanie, who did all the preliminary work on these cookies. Can you tell we all have a sweet tooth in my family?

Nutrition Information per Cookie

Calories	47.17
Protein	2.33 g
Carbs	3.44 g
Fat	3.06 g
Fiber	0.84 g
Net carb	2.60 g

DESSERTS

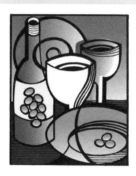

Almond Carrot Cake

....

1½ cups ground almonds
¾ cup finely grated carrot
1 tablespoon lemon zest
1 teaspoon ground ginger
½ teaspoon ground mace
½ teaspoon cinnamon
5 eggs, separated
11/4 cups granular Splenda
1 tablespoon baking powder
2 tablespoons Grand Marnier
2 tablespoons water
small amount of butter for pan
small amount of granular Splenda
Vanilla Custard Sauce (see recipe)

- Preheat oven to 350°.
- Lightly butter bottom and sides of a 10″ spring-form pan. Sprinkle with small amount of granular Splenda to coat and lightly tap to remove excess.
- In a mixing bowl, combine the spices with the ground almonds and mix well. Add the grated carrots and lemon zest and mix well. Set aside.
- In a deep bowl, beat the egg whites with an electric mixer until they form stiff peaks. (Do *not* use a stainless steel bowl since it will discolor the whites.)
- In a second deep bowl, using the same electric mixer, beat the egg yolks for about 30 seconds. Slowly sift the Splenda into the egg yolks and continue beating for another 3–4 minutes, until the yolks are pale yellow and thick.

continued

- With a wooden spoon, stir the baking powder, Grand Marnier, and water into the egg yolk mixture. Stir well, and this mixture will lighten in texture.
- Add the almond and carrot mixture to the egg mixture, in three equal parts, stirring to blend after each addition.
- Vigorously stir about ¼ of the egg whites into the carrot mixture to lighten it. Spoon the remaining egg whites into the carrot mixture and fold gently with a rubber spatula until no white streaks are left.
- Pour the batter into the prepared pan and bake for 50–60 minutes, until cake tests done with a toothpick.
- Cool on a wire rack for 10 minutes and then remove sides of pan. Cool completely.
- Serve thin wedges of cake with Vanilla Custard Sauce or a little whipped cream.

Makes 10 servings.

Nutrition Information per Serving	
Calories	139.84
Protein	6.64 g
Carbs	7.61 g
Fat	9.77 g
Fiber	2.03 g
Net carb	5.58 g

Baked Strawberries & Peaches

4 eggs
9 packets Splenda, divided
1⅓ cups heavy cream
1 teaspoon vanilla extract
2 tablespoons flour
2 peaches thinly sliced
1 cup sliced strawberries
½ teaspoon cinnamon

• Slice the peaches and strawberries and sprinkle with a mixture of 2 packets of Splenda and the cinnamon. Set aside.
• Preheat oven to 325°.
• Place the eggs, 7 packets of Splenda, and vanilla in a large bowl and beat with an electric mixer until frothy. Gradually sift the flour into the egg mixture and whisk to blend thoroughly.
• Pour ¾ of a cup of the egg mixture into a lightly greased 9″ pie plate. Bake for approximately 5 minutes, until the cream is just set.
• Remove the dish from the oven and spread the fruit evenly over the cream base. Pour the remaining cream mixture over the fruit and bake for 25–30 minutes or until completely set.
• Cool for 20 minutes before serving. May be served with a dollop of heavy cream that has been whipped with Splenda.
Makes 6–8 servings.

VARIATION: You may use other berries in place of the strawberries. The carb content will vary slightly.

Nutrition Information per Serving	
Calories	201.52
Protein	4.78 g
Carbs	8.08 g
Fat	16.92 g
Fiber	0.99 g
Net carb	7.09 g

Cherry Compote

⅔ cup red wine

1½ pounds fresh cherries

4 packets Splenda

½ teaspoon cinnamon

2 teaspoons cornstarch

- Wash and pit cherries. Set aside.
- Put red wine, cinnamon, and Splenda in a saucepan and heat over low heat for 2–3 minutes, until Splenda dissolves.
- Add the cherries and simmer for 6–8 minutes. Add some water if the wine does not cover the fruit. Remove from heat after 8 minutes.
- Dissolve cornstarch in a little water and add to the cherry mixture. Return to medium heat and bring to a boil, stirring constantly. The sauce will thicken into a syrup-like consistency.
- Transfer to a serving bowl or individual dessert bowls. May be served warm or cold.

Makes 8 servings.

NOTE: This is wonderful over a small dish of no-sugar-added vanilla ice cream, or low-carb vanilla ice cream, if you can afford the additional carbohydrates.

Nutrition Information per Serving

Calories	22.86
Protein	0.11 g
Carbs	2.38 g
Fat	0.08 g
Fiber	0.17 g
Net carb	2.21 g

Chocolate Almond Torte

4 squares semi-sweet baking chocolate (4 ounces), divided
4 squares bittersweet baking chocolate (4 ounces), divided
1 cup butter, divided
16 packets Splenda, divided
3 eggs
1 cup ground almonds
1 tablespoon orange zest
3 tablespoons heavy cream
toasted slivered almonds, to garnish
small amount of granular Splenda

- Preheat oven to 375°.
- Butter an 8″ round cake pan and line with parchment paper. Butter the parchment paper and sprinkle the sides and bottom of the pan with small amount of granular Splenda. Shake out excess.
- Melt the 2 squares each of the semi-sweet and bittersweet chocolate in the top of a double boiler. Set aside on a tea towel to cool slightly.
- Cream ¾ of a cup of the butter and 12 packets of Splenda (or ½ cup of granular Splenda) together with an electric mixer until fluffy. Add the eggs one at a time, beating well after each addition. With your beater on a low speed, add the chocolate and ground almonds. Stir in the orange zest.
- Pour the batter into the prepared pan. Bake for 20–25 minutes. The center will look soft, and the edges will look done.
- Remove to a cake rack and cool for 20 minutes. Using a small sharp knife, cut around the edges of the pan to release the cake. Invert the pan onto the rack. Peel off the parchment paper, turn cake right side up, and continue to cool for at least an hour.

continued

Glaze

- Melt the remaining chocolate, ¼ cup of butter, and 4 packets of Splenda in the top of a double boiler. Stir to blend while chocolate and butter melt. Cook until fully blended and smooth.
- Remove from heat and beat with a spoon to cool. Add the heavy cream while beating constantly.
- Place waxed paper under edges of cake on serving platter. Pour glaze over cake and allow it to run down the sides. Before glaze has cooled completely, press the toasted slivered almonds into a narrow band on the top of the cake as a decorative border. Gently pull the waxed paper from under the cake. If you like, omit the waxed paper and let the chocolate glaze drip onto the serving platter. *Makes 8 servings.*

Nutrition Information per Serving	
Calories	412.77
Protein	8.34 g
Carbs	12.80 g
Fat	42.21 g
Fiber	5.85 g
Net carb	6.95 g

Chocolate Indulgence

5 ounces unsweetened chocolate

5 ounces semi-sweet chocolate

1 cup unsalted butter

6 eggs

5 packets Splenda

1 tablespoon brandy extract

1 tablespoon flour

To Finish

1 cup heavy cream

4 packets Splenda

sprigs of fresh mint

1 cup fresh strawberries or raspberries

- Preheat oven to 350°.
- Grease a 9″ x 2″ round spring-form pan. Cut parchment paper for bottom and grease paper. Wrap the outside bottom and sides of the pan in tinfoil, to ensure it is completely watertight.
- In the top of a double boiler, melt chocolate and butter. This will be quicker if chocolate and butter are chopped into pieces. Add Splenda and stir until smooth.
- Remove from heat and let cool for 2–3 minutes. Set the top of the double boiler on a tea towel to absorb any moisture.
- Beat eggs in a large bowl with an electric beater for 1 minute. Add brandy extract and sifted flour and beat just to blend.

continued

- Gradually add chocolate mixture to egg mixture, beating slowly until completely blended. Pour into spring-form pan.
- Place spring-form pan in a roasting pan that has ½″ of water in the bottom. Place in the center of the oven and bake for 25–30 minutes, until the edges are set and the center is still soft.
- Remove from the oven. Gently remove tinfoil from around pan and place on a wire rack to cool for 15 minutes. The cake may sink in the center and may even crack, but don't be alarmed.
- Remove the cake from the spring-form pan; then place cake top down on wire rack to remove parchment paper. Let cool completely. You may decide that the bottom now becomes the top of the cake. I just pick whichever has the most pleasing appearance. This is a dense, heavy cake that is not very high.
- Move cake to a serving plate. Garnish with a light dusting of unsweetened cocoa, using a sifter to dust.
- To finish, slice a thin wedge of cake. Serve with a dollop of heavy cream whipped with Splenda, a sprig of fresh mint, and 2 or 3 fresh berries.

Makes 10 servings.

NOTE: The net carb content is low, but as with any rich chocolate dessert the calories are not. Just keep this in mind and save this cake for special occasions.

Nutrition Information per Serving

Calories	447.00
Protein	7.80 g
Carbs	10.07 g
Fat	45.90 g
Fiber	4.37 g
Net carb	5.70 g

Chocolate Mint Cake

Cake
½ cup oat flour
½ cup soy flour
⅓ cup unsweetened cocoa powder
½ teaspoon salt
¼ teaspoon baking soda
¼ teaspoon baking powder
¾ cup butter
12 packets Splenda
2 teaspoons vanilla extract
3 large eggs
½ cup light cream
1 cup miniature semi-sweet chocolate chips

Filling
1 cup semi-sweet chocolate chips
½ cup heavy cream
½ teaspoon peppermint extract

Frosting
6 ounces bittersweet chocolate
½ cup heavy cream
½ teaspoon peppermint extract

Garnish
small red & white mints (or small candy canes, crushed)

continued

Cake
- Preheat oven to 350°.
- Butter 2 round cake pans (8") and line with parchment paper. Butter the paper and up the sides of the pan and dust with oat flour.
- Bring the butter to room temperature. Whisk together the flour, cocoa powder, salt, baking powder, and baking soda until blended.
- With an electric mixer, beat butter until light and fluffy. Add the Splenda, then the vanilla and eggs, one at a time. Add the dry mixture, alternately with the cream, in two batches each, blending well after each addition. Mix in the chocolate chips.
- Pour the batter, evenly divided, into the 2 prepared cake pans. Smooth the batter in the pans until even. Bake in the center of the oven rack until tester inserted in the middle comes out clean. This will take approximately 40–45 minutes, depending on your oven.
- Cool on a cake rack for 5 minutes. Turn cake out onto a cooling rack, peel off the parchment, and cool completely.

Filling
- Place chocolate chips in a medium bowl.
- Bring cream to a simmer in a small saucepan.
- Pour the cream over the chocolate chips. Whisk to melt the chocolate and blend. Continue whisking until smooth. Add the peppermint extract and blend.
- Set aside to cool at room temperature while cakes cool.
- When you are ready to assemble (cakes should be completely cool throughout), beat the filling using the electric mixer until it is fluffy and light in color. This may take a few minutes.
- Place the bottom cake on a flat surface and examine the top to make sure it is flat. If necessary, slice a thin piece off the top to even it out. Spread the filling evenly over the top of this cake and place the second cake on top of the filling and gently press down to make sure that it is secure. Chill for 20 minutes before frosting.

continued

Frosting
- Cut the bittersweet chocolate into small pieces and place in a bowl.
- Bring the cream to a simmer in a small saucepan.
- Pour the cream over the chocolate pieces. Whisk to melt the chocolate and blend. Continue whisking until smooth and shiny. Add the peppermint extract and blend.
- Place the filled cake on a cake rack with waxed paper below the rack. Pour the frosting over the cake and let it run down the sides.

Garnish
- Put a few small red & white mints in the food processor and pulse for a couple of seconds to break them into small pieces. Sprinkle the mint pieces in a border around the top of the cake.

Makes 10 servings.

NOTE: This delicious cake has a high carb count, so I save it for very special occasions and have only a small piece — about half the serving size suggested by the recipe. It presents beautifully with the shiny chocolate frosting and the crushed candies.

Nutrition Information per Serving

Calories	476.26
Protein	8.34 g
Carbs	32.37 g
Fat	38.21 g
Fiber	2.17 g
Net carb	30.20 g

Chocolate Pavé

6 ounces unsweetened chocolate
4 ounces semi-sweet chocolate
½ cup unsalted butter
6 egg yolks
4 tablespoons heavy cream
4 packets Splenda

To Finish
½ cup heavy cream
2 packets Splenda
16–24 fresh cherries or
    raspberries

• Line a mini-loaf pan (2 cups) with two strips of waxed paper — one for the length and one for the width of the pan. Allow at least ½" to overhang on all sides. Set aside.
• In the top of a double boiler, melt the chocolate and butter. Add 4 packets of Splenda and stir until smooth. Set aside on a tea towel to cool for 2–3 minutes.
• In a large bowl, use a whisk to beat together egg yolks and the 4 tablespoons of heavy cream until smooth and creamy. Beat 2 or 3 spoonfuls of the chocolate mixture into the egg mixture. Gradually whisk the rest of the chocolate mixture into the egg mixture until completely blended.
• Pour into the loaf pan and let cool to room temperature. Place in the fridge for at least 3 hours.
• Remove the pavé by inverting the loaf pan. Peel off waxed paper and place on serving dish. Cut thin slices of the pavé and serve with a dollop of cream whipped with the Splenda and 2–3 fresh cherries or raspberries.

Makes 8 servings.

NOTE: This is a very rich, dark, and bitter-sweet chocolate dessert.

Nutrition Information per Serving	
Calories	369.03
Protein	5.13 g
Carbs	15.81 g
Fat	35.76 g
Fiber	3.27 g
Net carb	12.54 g

Chocolate Silk Pie

Crust

6 tablespoons butter

½ cup ground pecans

¾ cup ground almonds

6 tablespoons soy flour

¼ cup flax seed meal

1 teaspoon xanthan gum

4 packets Splenda

Filling

3 ounces unsweetened baking chocolate

1½ teaspoons vanilla extract

3 eggs

12 packets Splenda

¾ cup butter

Crust
- Preheat oven to 325°.
- Grind the pecans in a food processor or chop finely with a sharp knife.
- Mix all dry ingredients in a bowl.
- Melt the butter, add to the dry ingredients, and mix well. This will result in a crumble type of batter. Press evenly into a 9″ glass pie plate.
- Bake for 20 minutes, until golden brown.
- Place pie plate on a rack to cool.

continued

Filling
- Melt the chocolate in the top of a double boiler and set aside on a tea towel for a few minutes to cool.
- Cream butter and Splenda with an electric mixer until light and fluffy. With the mixer running at low speed, gradually add the chocolate and vanilla. Add the eggs one at a time, beating on medium speed for 5 minutes after each addition.
- Pour the filling into cooled pie crust and put in the fridge for 2–3 hours.
- Garnish with a small dollop of whipped cream or some fresh berries or a drizzle of chocolate sauce.

Makes 8 servings.

NOTE: This is a real indulgence because of the fat content — creamy, smooth, delicious, and worth the splurge!

Nutrition Information per Serving

Calories	458.97
Protein	9.51 g
Carbs	11.61 g
Fat	42.82 g
Fiber	3.80 g
Net carb	7.81 g

Crème Brûlée

2½ cups heavy cream
4 egg yolks
6 packets Splenda
1 teaspoon vanilla

- Preheat oven to 300°.
- Put the cream in the top of a double boiler over medium-high heat and, while stirring constantly, bring it to just below boiling. This will take about 5 minutes, and you will know it is ready when it starts to froth lightly.
- Put the egg yolks, Splenda, and vanilla extract in a mixing bowl and beat with an electric mixer for 2–3 minutes.
- Slowly add 2–3 tablespoons of the hot cream to the yolk mixture to temper it; then add the rest of the cream mixture and stir to combine.
- Pour the mixture into a shallow baking dish and place it in a roasting pan that has 1″ of water in the bottom. Bake at 300° for 45–60 minutes or until set (edges will be brown).
- Carefully remove the brûlée pan from the roasting pan and set on a tea towel to cool. Refrigerate until ready to serve. Serve with a garnish of fresh berries.
Makes 6 servings.

NOTE: This delicious dessert has everything except the burnt sugar coating you find on other brûlées.

Nutrition Information per Serving	
Calories	387.54
Protein	3.89 g
Carbs	4.05 g
Fat	40.11 g
Fiber	0.00 g
Net carb	4.05 g

Crème Brûlée with Raspberries

2½ cups heavy cream
4 egg yolks
6 packets Splenda

1 teaspoon vanilla
1 cup fresh raspberries (or
   frozen unsweetened)

- Preheat oven to 300°.
- Combine the egg yolks, Splenda, and vanilla in a separate bowl and beat with an electric mixer for 2 minutes. Set aside.
- Wash and pat dry the raspberries and set aside.
- Put cream in the top of a double boiler over medium heat and, stirring constantly, bring it to just below a boil. (The water in the bottom of the double boiler should be boiling lightly.) This will take about 5 minutes, and you will know that it is ready when it starts to froth lightly.
- Add a small amount of the hot cream (2–3 teaspoons) into the egg mixture and stir to temper the egg. Add the rest of the cream and stir to blend.
- Divide the custard evenly into 6 ramekins. Evenly divide the raspberries among the ramekins and gently drop into the custard. I try to place at least one raspberry so that it sits on top of the custard to add color. (If using frozen berries, they must be thawed before using.)
- Pour ½″ of water into a large roasting pan. Gently place the ramekins into the roasting pan, ensuring that no water gets into the custard.
- Bake for 35–40 minutes, until the custard is set in the middle and the edges are starting to brown.
- Carefully remove the ramekins from the roasting pan and set on a tea towel to cool. Refrigerate until serving time.

Makes 6 servings.

NOTE: This is a lovely creamy dessert, and the raspberries add a surprising taste treat.

Nutrition Information per Serving	
Calories	397.59
Protein	4.07 g
Carbs	6.42 g
Fat	40.22 g
Fiber	1.39 g
Net carb	5.03 g

Flourless Chocolate Cake

6 ounces bittersweet chocolate

2 ounces unsweetened chocolate

¼ pound butter

5 large eggs, separated

⅔ cup granular Splenda

- Preheat oven to 325°.
- Lightly grease an 8″ round pan and line the bottom with parchment paper.
- Melt chocolate and butter in the top of a double boiler, stirring occasionally. Allow to cool slightly.
- Whisk together the egg yolks and all but 3 tablespoons of the Splenda until you have a thick pale yellow mixture. Slowly add the cooled chocolate to the yolks.
- Beat the egg whites into stiff peaks, adding the remaining 3 tablespoons of Splenda as you beat them.
- Stir the chocolate mixture into the egg whites. Pour into the prepared pan and knock gently on the countertop to settle the air bubbles.
- Bake for 40–45 minutes or until toothpick comes out clean. Let cool on a wire rack for 5 minutes and then loosen cake around the edges and invert on a plate. Remove parchment covering, invert again on the rack, and let cool completely. *Cut into 8 wedges.*

PRESENTATION: You will find that this is a very rich cake. I like to serve it with a little whipped cream and a few fresh berries to help provide balance. I particularly like raspberries and blackberries. You could also serve on a berry purée or with a simple Chocolate Ganache (see recipe).

Thanks to Lynne Wilson of Lantzville, British Columbia, for this flourless cake.

Nutrition Information per Serving

Calories	300.39
Protein	6.56 g
Carbs	16.57 g
Fat	25.94 g
Fiber	2.71 g
Net carb	13.86 g

Julie's Middle Eastern Orange Cake

2 large oranges
6 eggs
1 cup granular Splenda

1½ cups ground almonds
1 teaspoon baking powder

- Wash and then simmer the whole oranges in water for 2 hours. Let cool. Quarter and remove any seeds. Place the sections (skins included) in a food processor or blender and process.
- Preheat oven to 375°.
- Line a 9″ spring-form pan with parchment paper.
- If you have a food processor, add all the remaining ingredients to the oranges and mix thoroughly. If you are using a blender, blend the oranges and eggs together, add them to the dry ingredients, and then mix well.
- Pour the batter into the prepared pan. Tap the pan gently on the countertop to even the batter.
- Bake for 50–60 minutes until the top of the cake is lightly browned. This cake does not rise, so it is fairly flat in the pan.
- Place on a wire rack to cool. Unmold the sides of the pan immediately and let cake cool for 10–15 minutes before taking the bottom part off. Cool completely before peeling the parchment paper off the cake.
- Serve with a drizzle of chocolate sauce or some fresh berries and whipped cream.

Makes 10 thin wedges.

NOTE: I have made this cake using 4 small tangerines in place of the oranges, and it was wonderful.

Thanks to Lynne Wilson of Lantzville, British Columbia, for this unusual and yummy cake.

Nutrition Information per Serving	
Calories	143.18
Protein	7.48 g
Carbs	8.99 g
Fat	10.25 g
Fiber	2.31 g
Net carb	6.68 g

Individual Chocolate Cakes

6 ounces bittersweet
  chocolate
½ cup butter
4 eggs
2 tablespoons prepared
  strong coffee

10 packets Splenda, divided
2 tablespoons flour
½ cup heavy cream
6 sprigs fresh mint

- Preheat oven to 400°.
- Spray 6 ramekins with a nonstick agent.
- Melt chocolate and butter in the top of a double boiler and stir to blend. Set aside.
- Beat eggs with coffee until foamy. Gradually add 8 packets of Splenda, one packet at a time, and continue beating until light and fluffy. Add flour and chocolate and beat at low speed until just blended.
- Fill each ramekin ¾ full with cake batter and place the ramekins on a cookie sheet.
- Bake for 12–15 minutes, until cakes are raised and a crust has formed over the top. Cool for at least 10 minutes.
- Whip the heavy cream with the 2 packets of Splenda until stiff peaks form.
- Invert cakes onto individual dessert plates and garnish with a dollop of whipped cream and a sprig of fresh mint. These cakes are best if served warm, but they may also be served at room temperature.

Makes 6 servings.

TIP: These cakes are lovely with a bit of Raspberry Purée placed on the bottom of the plate as additional garnish. The carbohydrate count is high, so I save them for special occasions and watch the content of the other dishes in the meal.

Nutrition Information per Serving

Calories	338.65
Protein	5.96 g
Carbs	18.90 g
Fat	26.70 g
Fiber	0.00 g
Net carb	18.90 g

Lemon Cream Pie

Crust
¾ cup flax seed meal
¾ cup ground almonds
4 tablespoons butter
5 packets Splenda
1 teaspoon xanthan gum

Filling
1 cup granulated Splenda, divided
4 eggs
½ cup fresh lemon juice (2–3 lemons)
1 cup heavy cream, divided

Crust
• Melt the butter. Mix the flax seed meal, ground almonds, xanthan gum, Splenda, and butter with a fork to blend well. This will make a sticky crumb mixture. Press into the bottom and up the sides of a 9″ glass pie plate.
• Bake at 375° for 10–12 minutes, until the edges are brown. Let cool completely.

Filling
• Take 2 teaspoons of zest from one of the lemons, wrap in plastic, and put in the fridge for use later. Squeeze ½ cup of fresh lemon juice.
• Whisk the eggs in a large bowl until fluffy. Gradually add ¾ cup of loose Splenda to the eggs. Whisk in the lemon juice and then gradually add ½ cup of the heavy cream.

continued

- Pour this lemon cream mixture into the pie plate and bake at 375° for 25–30 minutes or until the middle of the filling is set. Cool completely.
- To serve, whip the remaining heavy cream with the remaining Splenda and add the lemon rind to the whipped cream. Serve small wedges of pie with the lemon whipped cream on top.

Makes 8 servings.

Nutrition Information per Serving

Calories	299.79
Protein	8.37 g
Carbs	10.41 g
Fat	29.02 g
Fiber	4.11 g
Net carb	6.30 g

Lemon Custard Cake

2 large lemons
¼ cup flour
½ cup granular Splenda
3 eggs, separated
6 packets Splenda
1 cup whole milk
⅓ cup heavy cream

- Preheat oven to 350°.
- Finely grate the zest of 1 lemon, approximately 1 tablespoon. Squeeze 6 tablespoons of lemon juice from the lemons.
- Whisk together the flour, salt, and ½ cup of granular Splenda.
- Whisk together the yolks, milk, cream, lemon juice, and zest. Add to the flour mixture and stir until just combined.
- Beat the egg whites in a separate bowl until soft peaks form. Add 6 packets of Splenda, 2 at a time, until stiff peaks form and the egg whites are glossy.
- Whisk about ⅓ of the egg white mixture into the batter to lighten. Fold in the remaining egg white with a rubber spatula.
- Pour into a buttered 1½-quart shallow ceramic baking dish. Place this dish inside a roasting pan that has 1–2″ of water in the bottom. Bake until the cake is puffed and golden brown, about 40–50 minutes.
- Cool on a rack for a few minutes and serve warm. This great little cake may also be refrigerated and served again the following day.
Makes 6 servings.

Nutrition Information per Serving	
Calories	137.50
Protein	5.88 g
Carbs	12.27 g
Fat	8.93 g
Fiber	0.92 g
Net carb	11.35 g

Marinated Pineapple & Cherries

2 cups water
zest & juice of 1 lime
4 packets Splenda
½ teaspoon cinnamon
¼ cup sherry
½ pineapple
½–¾ pound fresh cherries

To Finish
1 cup heavy cream
2 packets Splenda
sprigs of fresh mint

• Put water, lime juice and zest, Splenda, cinnamon, and sherry in a heavy saucepan and bring to a simmer over medium heat. Reduce to a syrup-like consistency by simmering for approximately 30 minutes. Remove from heat and cool for 15 minutes.
• Cut off outer skin and hard core of pineapple and cut fruit into bite-sized pieces. Put pineapple chunks into a large bowl. Add cherries that have been washed and pitted (approximately 1 cup).
• Strain the cooled marinade and pour over the fruit. Put in the fridge for 2–3 hours, stirring occasionally.
• Whip the cream while gradually adding the Splenda until stiff peaks form.
• Spoon the fruit into individual dessert dishes. Finish with a dollop of whipped cream and a sprig of fresh mint.
Makes 8 servings.

Nutrition Information per Serving	
Calories	149.97
Protein	1.09 g
Carbs	10.62 g
Fat	11.42 g
Fiber	1.10 g
Net carb	9.52 g

Peach Cobbler

3 medium peaches (2½" diameter)

7 packets Splenda, divided

½ teaspoon ground cinnamon

⅛ teaspoon ground nutmeg

¾ cup almond slivers, roughly ground

⅓ cup oats

3 tablespoons butter

1 teaspoon xanthan gum

- Preheat oven to 375°.
- Cut butter into small pieces and let reach room temperature.
- Peel peaches and cut into bite-sized pieces. Mix peaches with 4 packets of Splenda and the cinnamon and nutmeg. Set aside for a few minutes.
- Mix the ground almonds, oats, butter, xanthan gum, and remaining 3 packets of Splenda. This will make a dry, crumbly topping. (I like to leave some of the almond pieces a little bigger to provide more crunch to the topping.)
- Lightly grease a 1½-quart ovenproof casserole dish. Pour peaches into the casserole and top with the oat mixture. Be sure to spread topping evenly and to the edges of the dish.
- Bake for 25 minutes, until the topping is browned and the fruit is bubbling. Let cool for 15 minutes.

Makes 6 servings.

NOTE: May be served with a small dollop of whipped cream or some light or low-carb vanilla ice cream.

Nutrition Information per Serving

Calories	179.74
Protein	4.40 g
Carbs	14.87 g
Fat	12.44 g
Fiber	3.41 g
Net carb	11.46 g

Peach Delight

½ cup fresh or frozen unsweetened raspberries
4 packets Splenda, divided
2 fresh peaches, peeled, pitted, and quartered
½ cup heavy cream
Raspberry Purée (see recipe)

• Whip the heavy cream with 2 packets of Splenda and set aside.
• Process the raspberries in a food processor with 2 packets of Splenda until smooth.
• Place the peach quarters on a broiler pan sprayed with a nonstick agent and place under a hot broiler until just brown, 2–3 minutes.
• Place 2 peach quarters in a dessert dish and drizzle with a generous portion of Raspberry Purée. Garnish with a dollop of whipped cream.
Makes 4 servings.

**Nutrition Information
per Serving**

Calories	145.93
Protein	1.24 g
Carbs	11.62 g
Fat	11.16 g
Fiber	2.05 g
Net carb	9.57 g

Peaches with Sweet Pecans

1 cup pecan halves
3 tablespoons butter
12 packets Splenda, divided
6 medium peaches (2½″ diameter)
½ cup heavy cream
¾ teaspoon cinnamon, divided

- Preheat oven to 375°.
- Melt 1 tablespoon of butter and mix with 4 packets of Splenda and ½ teaspoon of cinnamon.
- Line a baking pan with parchment paper. In a small bowl, toss pecans with the butter and spice mixture. Bake for 5 minutes, stir to turn nuts, and continue baking for another 10 minutes.
- Pour nuts onto a clean chopping board, let cool slightly, and chop roughly.
- Line pan with new parchment paper. Place peach halves in the pan. Melt the remaining tablespoon of butter and add 6 packets of Splenda and ¼ teaspoon of cinnamon. Brush the peach halves with this mixture and bake for 25–30 minutes until nicely browned on top.
- Place two peach halves on a dessert plate, sprinkle with roasted nuts, and top with a dollop of heavy cream whipped with 2 packets of Splenda.

Makes 6 servings, or serve 12 half peaches with the nuts and cream.

Nutrition Information per Serving	
Calories	286.09
Protein	2.80 g
Carbs	15.98 g
Fat	26.14 g
Fiber	3.73 g
Net carb	12.25 g

Pumpkin Custard

1½ cups heavy cream

12 packets Splenda

½ teaspoon rum extract

4 large egg yolks

1 cup canned pumpkin (not pie filling)

½ teaspoon cinnamon

¼ teaspoon nutmeg

¼ teaspoon ground cloves

⅛ teaspoon ground mace

⅛ teaspoon ground ginger

- Preheat oven to 325°.
- In a large saucepan, whisk together the cream, rum extract, spices, and Splenda. Heat over medium heat until steam rises and bubbles form around the edges. Remove from heat, whisking every minute or so to keep blended.
- In a large bowl, whisk the egg yolks until light and fluffy. Add pumpkin and whisk to blend. Very slowly add the warm cream mixture to the egg mixture until well blended.
- Pour into 6 small ramekins or individual custard cups. Fill a large roasting pan with ½″ of water and place the 6 dessert dishes in the water bath. Put the roasting pan in the oven and bake for 30–40 minutes, until just set. The mixture will appear slightly soft in the middle.
- Carefully remove ramekins from roasting pan, making sure not to get any water in the custards, and place on a wire rack to cool. Place in the fridge for 2–3 hours before serving. Serve with a small dollop of whipped cream.

Makes 6 servings.

Nutrition Information per Serving	
Calories	268.02
Protein	3.75 g
Carbs	27.28 g
Fat	25.46 g
Fiber	20.01 g
Net carb	7.27 g

Quick & Easy Mousse

1 small (1-ounce) Sugar Free Jell-O Instant Pudding mix
or (28-gram) package of Fat Free Jell-O Instant Pudding mix
1½ cups skim milk
½ cup heavy cream

• In a bowl, combine the pudding mix, skim milk, and heavy cream. Beat with an electric mixer for 2 minutes, until thickened.
• Pour or spoon into individual dessert dishes and refrigerate for at least 20 minutes, until set.
Makes 4 servings.

NOTE: What is called Sugar Free Jell-O Instant Pudding in the United States is marketed as Fat Free Jell-O Instant Pudding in Canada. It is essentially the same product.

TIP: This quick and easy dessert may be made using any flavor of Jell-O instant pudding mix. The grams of carbohydrate will vary slightly with the flavor of pudding. I used vanilla pudding mix to determine the nutritional information.

Nutrition Information per Serving

Calories	154.79
Protein	3.74 g
Carbs	10.29 g
Fat	11.17 g
Fiber	0.00 g
Net carb	10.29 g

Raspberries & Cream

1½ cups fresh or frozen raspberries
¾ cup heavy cream
2 packets Splenda
2 slices (¼") pound cake

Raspberry Sauce
juice of berries
2 teaspoons liqueur
¼ teaspoon xanthan gum

• This recipe works best with frozen, unsweetened raspberries. If you are using fresh raspberries, you will want to mash a few to make the purée.
• Thaw the berries and strain. Put berries in the fridge until needed. Take the liquid and place in a small saucepan. Add the liqueur (a fruit flavor works best) and the xanthan gum and whisk ingredients together. Turn the heat to medium and continue whisking while it cooks for 2–3 minutes. The sauce will thicken (due to the liqueur and the xanthan gum) as it cooks.
• Remove from heat and let cool. It will continue to thicken as it cools. If your sauce gets too thick to pour, you can thin it a bit with water.
• Whip the heavy cream with the Splenda until fairly stiff.
• Cut the two slices of pound cake into small cubes.
• Assemble just an hour before serving, or the whipped cream breaks down. Keep in the fridge until ready to serve. You can assemble in four glass dessert dishes, but I particularly like the appearance when it is assembled in a martini glass.

continued

- Evenly divide the cake cubes among the four dishes and place them in the bottom. They do not need to be even or flat. Pour the raspberry sauce over the cake and let it run down the sides of the dish. Spoon a little of the whipped cream over the drenched cake. Divide the berries evenly among the dishes, reserving one raspberry as garnish for each dish. Spoon the remaining whipped cream over the berries, reaching to the edge of the dish if possible. Place a single berry on top of each dish.
- This is a delicious dessert that is beautiful to look at due to the layered effect of the berries and cream.

Makes 4 servings.

NOTE: I usually don't use all the raspberry sauce when I assemble this dessert. Any extra sauce can be served over low-carb ice cream or any other small treat the following day.

Nutrition Information per Serving

Calories	182.24
Protein	1.53 g
Carbs	13.17 g
Fat	14.26 g
Fiber	3.14 g
Net carb	10.03 g

Raspberry Cheesecake

Crust
1 cup pecan pieces (or walnut)
1 cup almond pieces
2 packets Splenda
1 teaspoon xanthan gum
2 tablespoons melted butter

Filling
2 packages (250 grams each) light cream cheese
2 packages (250 grams each) cream cheese
4 large eggs
¼ cup heavy cream
2 teaspoons vanilla extract
10 packets Splenda

Topping
2 cups fresh (or frozen, unsweetened) raspberries
4 packets Splenda
4 teaspoons lemon juice

• Preheat oven to 325°.
• Butter a 9″ spring-form pan and set aside.
• Finely chop the nuts or put in a food processor and pulse for about 10 seconds. You do not want the nuts to be powdered but finely chopped. Add the melted butter, xanthan gum, nuts, and Splenda and mix well. Press the crust into the pan and bake for 10–12 minutes or until lightly browned. Remove from the oven and let cool.

continued

- Allow the cream cheese to come to room temperature and beat with an electric mixer until smooth. This is easier to do if you chop the cream cheese into pieces before beating. Add the Splenda and continue beating. Add the eggs one at a time and beat the mixture after each egg. Add the heavy cream and vanilla extract and beat well to mix all ingredients.
- Pour the cheese mixture into the spring-form pan and even out the top with a spatula.
- Put the raspberries, lemon juice, and Splenda into a blender or food processor and purée. (If using frozen berries, they must be completely thawed before blending.) You may strain the purée if you don't like the seeds.
- Using approximately ¼ of the raspberry purée, drop it by spoonfuls on top of the cheese mixture, distributing the spoonfuls around the perimeter of the pan. Using a sharp knife, "cut" into the raspberry purée dollops and drag out to points. Do this 2 or 3 times for each dollop of raspberry, making an attractive pattern on top of the cake.
- Place the pan in the middle of the oven and bake for 55–60 minutes, until set and slightly brown at the edges. Remove from the oven and place on a cookie rack to cool.
- After about 10 minutes, take a sharp knife and run the blade around the perimeter before loosening the sides of the pan. Let the cheesecake cool completely and then place it in the fridge until serving time. I do not try to take the cake off the bottom of the spring form. If I want to take the cheesecake to the table to serve, I just place the spring-form bottom on an attractive serving plate.
- To serve, place a piece of cheesecake on a dessert plate and drizzle the plate with the remaining raspberry purée. This is easiest to do with a small squeeze bottle sold in kitchen and dollar stores.

Makes 10–12 servings.

NOTE: This cheesecake presents beautifully for a special occasion with its red raspberry top and garnish. I have had guests tell me that it was the best cheesecake they ever tasted!

Nutrition Information per Serving	
Calories	415.49
Protein	11.56 g
Carbs	8.64 g
Fat	39.09 g
Fiber	1.62 g
Net carb	7.02 g

Rhubarb & Strawberry Supreme

3 cups fresh rhubarb, cut into 1″ pieces
2 cups fresh strawberries, cut into halves or quarters
1/3 cup water
4 packets Splenda
1 teaspoon lemon juice

To Finish
1 cup heavy cream
2 packets Splenda
½ cup toasted almond slivers

• Put water, rhubarb, and Splenda into saucepan and heat over medium heat until water simmers. Lower heat and simmer for 5 minutes. Add strawberry pieces and continue to simmer for 2–3 minutes. Remove from heat and let cool.
• To serve, whip the cream with Splenda until stiff peaks form. Place rhubarb & strawberry mixture into individual dessert dishes and garnish with a dollop of whipped cream and a sprinkle of toasted almond slivers.
Makes 8 servings.

Nutrition Information per Serving	
Calories	169.30
Protein	2.76 g
Carbs	7.63 g
Fat	14.99 g
Fiber	2.45 g
Net carb	5.18 g

Strawberries Dipped in Chocolate

12 medium strawberries
2 ounces unsweetened chocolate
8 packets Splenda

- Wash and pat dry strawberries, leaving stems intact. Set aside.
- Melt chocolate in the top of a double boiler. Stir until smooth. Add the Splenda and continue stirring until dissolved. Remove top of double boiler from the heat and set on a kitchen towel.
- Holding berry by the green stem, dip it on both sides into the chocolate. You may want to scrape any excess off one side of the berry on the side of the double boiler.
- Set the berry down on a small cookie sheet covered with waxed paper. When all the berries have been dipped, put the cookie sheet in the fridge to set the chocolate. Berries should stay in the fridge until ready to serve.
- They can be prepared half a day ahead, but the berry will start to shrink inside the chocolate coating after a day.

Makes 12 servings.

NOTE: You will need sweet, ripe berries for this treat. The chocolate tastes like a dark bittersweet coating.

VARIATION: An alternative would be to melt a couple of the Lindt 70% Cocoa Dark Chocolate bars in the top of the double boiler and just dip the strawberries. This will be a bit higher in carbs.

Nutrition Information per Serving

Calories	30.93
Protein	0.56 g
Carbs	2.85 g
Fat	2.66 g
Fiber	1.00 g
Net carb	1.85 g

Strawberry Mousse

1 small package (8.5 grams) Strawberry Sugar Free Jell-O
or 1 small package (11.2 grams) Light Jell-O
⅔ cup boiling water
1 cup ice cubes
1 cup heavy cream
2 packets Splenda
1 cup finely cut-up fresh strawberries

• Whip the heavy cream with the Splenda until fairly stiff and set aside.
• In a large bowl, dissolve the Jell-O powder in the boiling water and stir for 2 minutes, until completely dissolved. Add the ice cubes and stir until the mixture begins to thicken, approximately 2–3 minutes. Remove any remaining unmelted ice cubes.
• Add the whipped cream and whisk gently to combine. Fold in the fruit.
• Spoon into individual dessert dishes and refrigerate for at least 30 minutes, until set.
Makes 6 servings.

TIP: A similar dessert may be made using Raspberry Jell-O and fresh raspberries.

NOTE: What is called Sugar Free Jell-O in the United States is marketed as Light Jell-O in Canada. It is essentially the same product.

VARIATION: You can pour the mousse into an attractive serving dish and let it set in the fridge. If you are bringing the dish to the table to serve, thinly slice a few strawberries to garnish the top. This recipe doubles well.

Nutrition Information per Serving	
Calories	147.73
Protein	1.15 g
Carbs	3.38 g
Fat	14.78 g
Fiber	0.64 g
Net carb	2.74 g

Strawberry Rhubarb Crumble

Filling
1 cup ¼″ pieces fresh rhubarb
1 cup cut-up fresh strawberries
    (4 large or 8 medium berries)
2 packets Splenda

Topping
¼ cup rolled oats (not the
    instant variety)
¼ cup finely chopped pecans
1 tablespoon butter at room
    temperature
1 teaspoon xanthan gum
2 packets Splenda

To Finish
½ cup heavy cream
2 packets Splenda
fresh mint sprigs
Whipped Cream (see recipe)

- Preheat oven to 375°.
- Mix together filling ingredients in a bowl and set aside. Mix together topping ingredients until crumbly mixture forms.
- Grease 4 small ramekins. Divide fruit mixture equally among ramekins. Sprinkle oat and nut mixture evenly on top of fruit, covering as much of the fruit as possible. Place ramekins on cookie sheet and bake for 25 minutes or until tops are browned and fruit is bubbling.
- Cool at least 30 minutes before serving. Garnish with a dollop of Whipped Cream (see recipe) and a sprig of fresh mint.
Makes 4 servings.

Nutrition Information per Serving	
Calories	131.27
Protein	2.88 g
Carbs	12.79 g
Fat	8.40 g
Fiber	3.25 g
Net carb	9.54 g

Stewed Rhubarb

3 cups fresh rhubarb, cut into 1″ pieces
¼ cup water
4 packets Splenda
1 teaspoon lemon juice

To Finish
½ cup heavy cream
2 packets Splenda
fresh mint sprigs

• Put water, lemon juice, rhubarb, and Splenda into saucepan and heat over medium heat until water simmers. Lower heat and simmer for 10 minutes. Remove from heat and let cool.
• To serve, whip the cream with Splenda until stiff peaks form. Place rhubarb in individual dessert dishes and garnish with a dollop of whipped cream and a sprig of fresh mint.
Makes 4 servings.

NOTE: If you are feeling indulgent, this is a wonderful topping for a light vanilla ice cream. The new low-carb ice creams are also wonderful with this as a topping. No need for the whipped cream in this case.

Nutrition Information per Serving

Calories	122.12
Protein	1.44 g
Carbs	6.57 g
Fat	11.19 g
Fiber	1.65 g
Net carb	4.92 g

Warm Chocolate Cakes

4 ounces bittersweet chocolate

½ cup butter, roughly chopped

2 large eggs

2 egg yolks

4 packets Splenda

2 tablespoons flour

To Finish

Raspberry Purée (see recipe)

Whipped Cream (see recipe)

- Preheat oven to 350°.
- Butter 6 ramekins or custard cups.
- Put chocolate and butter pieces in the top of a double boiler with hot water in the bottom, over medium heat. Stir until melted and well blended. Remove from heat and cool.
- Using an electric mixer, beat eggs, egg yolks, and Splenda until thick and pale yellow, about 5 minutes.
- Fold cooled chocolate into egg mixture. Sift flour into chocolate and fold until just blended.
- Divide the mixture evenly among the prepared dishes and place them on a cookie sheet. Bake until the edges are set, but cakes are still soft in the middle, approximately 15–18 minutes.
- Serve warm with a drizzle of Raspberry Purée and a dollop of Whipped Cream (see recipe).

Makes 6 servings.

Nutrition Information per Serving	
Calories	341.53
Protein	5.29 g
Carbs	10.81 g
Fat	34.46 g
Fiber	0.70 g
Net carb	10.11 g

Warm Spicy Peaches

2 tablespoons butter
2 packets Splenda
1 teaspoon vanilla extract
¼ teaspoon ground cardamom
¼ teaspoon ground nutmeg
4 ripe medium peaches

To Finish
½ cup heavy cream
2 packets Splenda

- Clean, skin, and pit peaches. Cut into ¼" thick slices and set aside.
- Melt butter in a large frying pan over medium heat. Add Splenda and stir until dissolved. Add spices and stir for 1 or 2 minutes.
- Add peaches and stir for approximately 5 minutes, turning occasionally to coat all sides.
- Whip heavy cream with the Splenda, until stiff peaks form.
- Serve peaches in individual dessert dishes with a dollop of whipped cream on top.

Makes 4 servings.

TIP: The peaches may be prepared earlier, up to a couple of hours before the meal, and gently reheated just before serving. They are best if served just warm, with the cool whipped cream.

**Nutrition Information
per Serving**

Calories	90.92
Protein	0.64 g
Carbs	9.56 g
Fat	5.88 g
Fiber	1.64 g
Net carb	7.92 g

Warm Spicy Strawberries

2 cups sliced strawberries
4 packets Splenda, divided
½ teaspoon cinnamon

- Slice the strawberries and sprinkle with a mixture of Splenda and the cinnamon.
- Microwave the fruit for 30 seconds at high power. Stir to blend. Microwave a second time for 20 seconds and stir well. Let the berries sit for approximately 20 minutes. Just before serving, microwave for 10 seconds to reheat.
- Serve warm with a dollop of whipped cream, over some low-carb ice cream, or just as is.

Makes 4 servings.

Nutrition Information per Serving

Calories	27.16
Protein	0.46 g
Carbs	6.50g
Fat	0.28 g
Fiber	1.87 g
Net carb	4.63 g

Warm Strawberries with Peaches

2 peaches, thinly sliced
1 cup sliced strawberries
4 packets Splenda, divided
1 teaspoon cinnamon

• Slice the peaches and strawberries and sprinkle with a mixture of Splenda and cinnamon.
• Microwave the fruit for 30 seconds at high power. Stir to blend. Microwave a second time for 20 seconds and stir well. Let the fruit sit for approximately 20 minutes. Just before serving, microwave for 10 seconds to reheat.
• Serve warm with a dollop of whipped cream, over some low-carb ice cream, or just as is.
Makes 4 servings.

VARIATION: You may use other berries in place of the strawberries. The carb content will vary slightly.

Nutrition Information per Serving	
Calories	48.59
Protein	0.81 g
Carbs	11.93 g
Fat	0.32 g
Fiber	2.85 g
Net carb	9.08 g

White Chocolate Mousse

1 small package (1 ounce) Sugar Free White Chocolate Jell-O
instant pudding mix
1½ cups skim milk
1 cup + ½ cup heavy cream
2 packets Splenda
fresh strawberries or raspberries, to garnish

• Whip 1 cup of the heavy cream with the Splenda until stiff peaks form.
• In another bowl, add Jell-O powder, milk, and remaining heavy cream and
whisk by hand for 2–3 minutes, until pudding starts to thicken.
• Add the whipped cream and whisk gently until well blended. Spoon into
individual dessert dishes and place in the fridge for 25–30 minutes.
• Garnish with fresh fruit cut into thin slices and placed on top of mousse.
Makes 6 servings.

NOTE: What is called Sugar Free Jell-O
Instant Pudding in the United States is mar-
keted as Fat Free Jell-O Instant Pudding in
Canada. It is essentially the same product.

**Nutrition Information
per Serving**

Calories	236.61
Protein	3.72 g
Carbs	6.41 g
Fat	22.27 g
Fiber	0.00 g
Net carb	6.41 g

White & Dark Chocolate Mousse

....

200 grams Lindt White Chocolate
200 grams Lindt 70% Cocoa Dark Chocolate
2½ cups heavy cream, divided

• Melt the white and dark chocolate separately in tops of double boilers. Set aside on tea towels to cool slightly.
• Divide the heavy cream into two equal portions of 1¼ cups each. In separate bowls, whip the cream just to the soft-peak stage.
• Fold the chocolate separately into each cream mixture using a rubber spatula. You will have a bowl of white chocolate mousse and another bowl of dark chocolate mousse. You may either place each mousse into a separate pasty bag or use a spoon to finish.
• Layer the white and dark mousse into an attractive serving bowl or into martini glasses. Place in the fridge to chill for 2–3 hours. Garnish with a few fresh berries.

Makes 8 servings.

NOTE: This is another indulgence, but it is absolutely gorgeous to look at in clear martini glasses, and it tastes wonderful. Save this dessert for those special occasions.

Thanks to Monique Coyle, who inspired me to develop this dish. She received the original version of this recipe from the chef at the Royal Colwood Golf and Country Club in Victoria, British Columbia.

Nutrition Information per Serving

Calories	537.84
Protein	5.27 g
Carbs	23.95 g
Fat	46.48 g
Fiber	1.25 g
Net carb	22.70 g